Population Health in Challenging Environments

Insights from Key Domains

PROCEEDINGS OF A WORKSHOP

Alina B. Baciu, *Rapporteur*

Roundtable on Population Health Improvement

Board on Population Health and Public Health Practice

Health and Medicine Division

The National Academies of
SCIENCES · ENGINEERING · MEDICINE

THE NATIONAL ACADEMIES PRESS
Washington, DC
www.nap.edu

THE NATIONAL ACADEMIES PRESS   500 Fifth Street, NW   Washington, DC 20001

This activity was supported by contracts between the National Academy of Sciences and the Association of American Medical Colleges, Aetna Foundation, Blue Cross Blue Shield of North Carolina, Blue Shield of California Foundation, The California Endowment, Geisinger, Jefferson University, The Kresge Foundation, National Association of County and City Health Officials, Nemours, New York State Health Foundation, The Rippel Foundation, Robert Wood Johnson Foundation, Samueli Foundation, The University of Texas at Austin, and Wake Forest Baptist Health. Any opinions, findings, conclusions, or recommendations expressed in this publication do not necessarily reflect the views of any organization or agency that provided support for the project.

International Standard Book Number-13: 978-0-309-46927-2
International Standard Book Number-10: 0-309-46927-9
Digital Object Identifier: https://doi.org/10.17226/26143

Additional copies of this publication are available from the National Academies Press, 500 Fifth Street, NW, Keck 360, Washington, DC 20001; (800) 624-6242 or (202) 334-3313; http://www.nap.edu.

Printed in the United States of America

Suggested citation: National Academies of Sciences, Engineering, and Medicine. 2023. *Population health in challenging times: Insights from key domains: Proceedings of a workshop*. Washington, DC: The National Academies Press. https://doi.org/10.17226/26143.

The National Academies of
SCIENCES · ENGINEERING · MEDICINE

The **National Academy of Sciences** was established in 1863 by an Act of Congress, signed by President Lincoln, as a private, nongovernmental institution to advise the nation on issues related to science and technology. Members are elected by their peers for outstanding contributions to research. Dr. Marcia McNutt is president.

The **National Academy of Engineering** was established in 1964 under the charter of the National Academy of Sciences to bring the practices of engineering to advising the nation. Members are elected by their peers for extraordinary contributions to engineering. Dr. John L. Anderson is president.

The **National Academy of Medicine** (formerly the Institute of Medicine) was established in 1970 under the charter of the National Academy of Sciences to advise the nation on medical and health issues. Members are elected by their peers for distinguished contributions to medicine and health. Dr. Victor J. Dzau is president.

The three Academies work together as the **National Academies of Sciences, Engineering, and Medicine** to provide independent, objective analysis and advice to the nation and conduct other activities to solve complex problems and inform public policy decisions. The National Academies also encourage education and research, recognize outstanding contributions to knowledge, and increase public understanding in matters of science, engineering, and medicine.

Learn more about the National Academies of Sciences, Engineering, and Medicine at **www.nationalacademies.org**.

The National Academies of
SCIENCES · ENGINEERING · MEDICINE

PLANNING COMMITTEE ON POPULATION HEALTH IN CHALLENGING TIMES: INSIGHTS FROM KEY DOMAINS[1]

SANNE MAGNAN (*Chair*), Senior Fellow, HealthPartners Institute
JOHN AUERBACH, Executive Director, Trust for America's Health
BOBBY MILSTEIN, Director, ReThink Health
LOURDES J. RODRIGUEZ, Senior Program Officer, St. David's Foundation

---

[1] The planning committee's role was limited to planning the workshop, and the Proceedings of a Workshop was prepared by the workshop rapporteur as a factual summary of what occurred at the workshop. Statements, recommendations, and opinions expressed are those of individual presenters and participants, and are not necessarily endorsed or verified by the National Academies of Sciences, Engineering, and Medicine, and they should not be construed as reflecting any group consensus.

ROUNDTABLE ON POPULATION HEALTH IMPROVEMENT[1]

SANNE MAGNAN (*Co-Chair*), Senior Fellow, HealthPartners Institute

JOSHUA M. SHARFSTEIN (*Co-Chair*), Vice Dean for Public Health Practice and Community Engagement, Professor of the Practice, Johns Hopkins Bloomberg School of Public Health

PHILIP M. ALBERTI, Senior Director, Health Equity Research and Policy, Association of American Medical Colleges

DAWN ALLEY, Chief Strategy Officer, Center for Medicare & Medicaid Innovation, Centers for Medicare & Medicaid Services

JOHN AUERBACH, Executive Director, Trust for America's Health

CATHY BAASE, Chair, Board of Directors, Michigan Health Improvement Alliance; Consultant for Health Strategy, The Dow Chemical Company

RAYMOND BAXTER, Trustee, Blue Shield of California Foundation

DEBBIE I. CHANG, President and Chief Executive Officer, Blue Shield of California Foundation

ALLISON GERTEL-ROSENBERG, Operational Vice President, National Policy and Practice, Nemours

MARC N. GOUREVITCH, Professor and Chair, Department of Population Health, New York University Langone Health

GARTH GRAHAM, President, Aetna Foundation

MARGARET GUERIN-CALVERT, Senior Managing Director and President, Center for Healthcare, Economics and Policy, FTI Consulting

GARY R. GUNDERSON, Vice President, Faith Health, School of Divinity, Wake Forest University

DORA HUGHES, Associate Research Professor of Health Policy and Management, Milken Institute School of Public Health, The George Washington University

SHERI JOHNSON, Director, Population Health Institute; Acting Director, Robert Wood Johnson Foundation Culture of Health Prize; Associate Professor, Department of Population Health Sciences, School of Medicine and Public Health, University of Wisconsin–Madison

WAYNE JONAS, Executive Director, Integrative Health Programs, H&S Ventures, Samueli Foundation

---

[1] The National Academies of Sciences, Engineering, and Medicines planning committees are solely responsible for organizing the workshop, identifying topics, and choosing speakers. The responsibility for the published Proceedings of a Workshop rests with the workshop rapporteur and the institution.

Reviewers

This Proceedings of a Workshop was reviewed in draft form by individuals chosen for their diverse perspectives and technical expertise. The purpose of this independent review is to provide candid and critical comments that will assist the National Academies of Sciences, Engineering, and Medicine in making each published proceedings as sound as possible and to ensure that it meets the institutional standards for quality, objectivity, evidence, and responsiveness to the charge. The review comments and draft manuscript remain confidential to protect the integrity of the process.

We thank the following individuals for their review of this proceedings:

RAYMOND BAXTER, Blue Shield of California Foundation
MARGARET GUERIN-CALVERT, FTI Consulting

Although the reviewers listed above provided many constructive comments and suggestions, they were not asked to endorse the content of the proceedings nor did they see the final draft before its release. The review of this proceedings was overseen by **GEORGE J. ISHAM,** HealthPartners Institute. He was responsible for making certain that an independent examination of this proceedings was carried out in accordance with standards of the National Academies and that all review comments were carefully considered. Responsibility for the final content rests entirely with the rapporteur and the National Academies. We also thank staff member **ALEXANDRA BEATTY** for reading and providing helpful comments on this manuscript.

Contents

Acronyms and Abbreviations

AAMC	Association of American Medical Colleges
CARES Act	2020 Coronavirus Aid, Relief, and Economic Security Act
CDC	Centers for Disease Control and Prevention
CHW	community health worker
CMS	Centers for Medicare & Medicaid Services
ESG	environmental, social, and governance
FQHC	federally qualified health center
GHPC	Georgia Health Policy Center
NQF	National Quality Forum
NYU	New York University
PRI	program-related investment
UCSF	University of California, San Francisco
WE in the World	Well-being and Equity in the World
WIN	Well Being In the Nation

1

Introduction

The year 2020 presented extraordinary challenges to organizations working to improve population health—from public health agencies at all levels of government to health systems to community-based non-profit organizations working to respond to health-related social needs. Between September 21 and 24, 2020, the Roundtable on Population Health Improvement held a workshop in six online sessions titled Population Health in Challenging Times: Insights from Key Domains. The concept for the workshop arose from a growing need to understand how the different domains in the population health field are responding to and being changed by the two major crises that they are confronting—racial injustice and the COVID-19 pandemic—within the societal context that also includes the national opioid overdose "epidemic" and other challenges. The workshop was organized by a planning committee composed of members of the Roundtable on Population Health Improvement: Sanne Magnan (*Chair*), John Auerbach, Bobby Milstein, and Lourdes Rodriguez. The charge to the planning committee is described in Box 1-1, and the workshop sessions were organized around five key domains:

1. Academic public health and population health,
2. The social sector,
3. Health care,
4. Governmental public health, and
5. Philanthropy.

A sixth session showcased high-level themes in cross-sector work. Each panel was designed to bring together several individuals with deep knowledge of that domain who were able to clearly articulate difficulties and opportunities, both internal and external, to their organizations.

Since February 2013, the Roundtable on Population Health Improvement has provided a trusted venue for leaders from the public and private sectors to meet and discuss leverage points and opportunities arising from changes in the social and political environment for achieving better population health. Population health is defined by Kindig and Stoddart (2003) as the health outcomes of a population, the patterns of determinants that shape those outcomes, and the interventions, including policies and investments, that link outcomes and determinants.

The roundtable's vision is of a thriving, healthful, and equitable society. The roundtable describes its mission as follows:

> In recognition that health and quality of life for all are shaped by interdependent historical and contemporary social, political, economic, environmental, genetic, behavioral, and health care factors, the roundtable exists to provoke and catalyze urgently needed multisector community-engaged collaborative action.[1]

In his introductory remarks orienting viewers to the week's sessions, Joshua Sharfstein, vice dean at the Johns Hopkins University Bloomberg School of Public Health, roundtable co-chair, and moderator of the first session and panel, noted that each of the conversations expected to take place throughout the workshop would be "anchored in the incredible moment in time we are finding ourselves in." He went on to note how the pandemic has "revealed profound inequities in our society and societies all around the world, most recently with the startling statistic" that more

---

BOX 1-1
Statement of Task

A planning committee of the National Academies of Sciences, Engineering, and Medicine will organize a workshop that will explore and highlight insights, current efforts, and ideas for the future in the field of population health improvement, which is experiencing a public health emergency along with other challenges and threats. The workshop will concentrate on key domains, such as government public health, nonprofit, philanthropy, health care, and cross-sector partnerships. Presentations and dialogue may be structured around the topics of measurement, policy, research, resources, communication, and cross-sector relationships. A proceedings summarizing the presentations and discussions at the workshop will be prepared by a designated rapporteur in accordance with institutional guidelines.

---

[1] See http://nas.edu/pophealthrt (accessed June 23, 2021).

than 75 percent of children who have died from COVID-19 are from communities of color. The pandemic is intertwined, he noted, with

> the crisis that reflects the exposure of racism in our society, the murder of [George] Floyd, the protest that followed, and the recognition that it is not just law enforcement that has a reckoning with race but many other fields including health and population health as well.

Sharfstein then enumerated the other crises affecting the health of American communities, from the overdose crisis, which is likely worsening during the pandemic, to the growing food insecurity affecting so many families around the country. Sharfstein stated that

> This is an extraordinary time for the country and an extraordinary time for our field ... and the discussions that will happen this week are going to be about what each of these domains can do to rise to the moment, to respond to the crises, and to provide greater vision and support for the country and the world moving forward.

This Proceedings of a Workshop summarizes remarks and conversations from the six distinct panels listed above from Chapters 2 to 7: academia, the social sector, health care, (governmental) public health, philanthropy, and cross-sector partnerships. Each panel offered a compelling mix of introspection and ideas to further the role and influence of its sector in nurturing the conditions for equitable health and well-being in communities during the pandemic, recovery, and into the future. Highlights from the remarks and discussions are summarized in Box 1-2.

BOX 1-2
Highlights from the Workshop

- Individual speakers from each panel reflected on the steps, including difficult work, infrastructure building, and systemic changes, that their sector needs to make internally, within organizations, and outwardly facing in their relationships with communities and other sectors and peers in order to respond to the crises of the pandemic and racial injustice.
- Authentically engaging and partnering with communities and sharing power with them requires listening, respecting, and integrating lived experience in the work of population health improvement. (Gunderson, Kangovi, Saha, and others)
- The crises of 2020—the movement against racial injustice, the COVID-19 pandemic, and the inequities it has laid bare—are not new. They are grounded in history and in structural and systemic factors. (Alberti, Khaldun, Parker, Purnell, Whitney-West, and others)
- Questions about the role of the public sector and government (especially federal and state governments) in coordination, funding, measurement, and other areas will need to be addressed as society and different sectors work to end the pandemic and to further racial justice. (Dreyfus, Hughes, and others)

2

Academic Public Health and Population Health

Joshua Sharfstein introduced the panelists, all of whom were drawn from schools and programs in public health and population health. He first invited them to share their thoughts about what academia can do at this moment of crisis for the field and the nation, both in terms of how institutions respond to crises in partnership with communities and other sectors, and how they transform their internal structure, culture, and processes. Key points from the panelists are provided in Box 2-1.

Dora Hughes from The George Washington University Milken Institute School of Public Health began her remarks with a quote from James Baldwin: "Not everything that is faced can be changed, but nothing can be changed until it is faced." The current crises—and in addition to those outlined in the introduction, she included wildfires, floods, and climate change more broadly—reveal the consequences of not facing or acknowledging key public health issues such as "avoidable, unfair, and remediable differences in health." She highlighted three key roles for academia in times of a public health crisis: advocacy for science and transparency, supporting or facilitating coordination on the marshalling of data and evidence in responding to the crisis, and providing support for governmental public health officials.

Regarding the first role, Hughes offered a specific example of lack of transparency: the delay on the part of the Centers for Disease Control and Prevention (CDC) in reporting demographic data that it was gathering about the pandemic's disproportionate impact on Black, Latino, and low-income populations. She noted that the void of federal data was filled in by data and analyses from universities, adding that reliance on academic

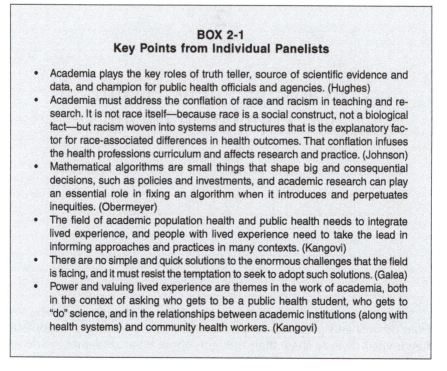

BOX 2-1
Key Points from Individual Panelists

- Academia plays the key roles of truth teller, source of scientific evidence and data, and champion for public health officials and agencies. (Hughes)
- Academia must address the conflation of race and racism in teaching and research. It is not race itself—because race is a social construct, not a biological fact—but racism woven into systems and structures that is the explanatory factor for race-associated differences in health outcomes. That conflation infuses the health professions curriculum and affects research and practice. (Johnson)
- Mathematical algorithms are small things that shape big and consequential decisions, such as policies and investments, and academic research can play an essential role in fixing an algorithm when it introduces and perpetuates inequities. (Obermeyer)
- The field of academic population health and public health needs to integrate lived experience, and people with lived experience need to take the lead in informing approaches and practices in many contexts. (Kangovi)
- There are no simple and quick solutions to the enormous challenges that the field is facing, and it must resist the temptation to seek to adopt such solutions. (Galea)
- Power and valuing lived experience are themes in the work of academia, both in the context of asking who gets to be a public health student, who gets to "do" science, and in the relationships between academic institutions (along with health systems) and community health workers. (Kangovi)

partners to highlight a data gap was not unprecedented. Her university, she stated, had determined the accurate number of casualties from Hurricane Maria in 2017—an effort that ultimately helped replace Puerto Rico's official total death toll of 64 with an estimate of nearly 3,000 deaths, and was followed by a commitment from the territory's government to improve its preparedness and response capabilities.

The second role for academia, Hughes remarked, is that its dedication to teaching, research, and service ought to include advocacy for science and transparency. An additional role of academia in a public health crisis is to facilitate and develop an infrastructure for coordination and collaboration, perhaps under the auspices of public health organizations.

A third potential role for academia, Hughes asserted, in a similar vein to what she called truth telling about science and evidence, is supporting and providing cover for public health officials operating on the front lines of a crisis. Hughes made note of the 49 public health leaders who resigned or were fired during the unfolding pandemic.[1] Sharfstein agreed, stating that public health leaders in academia do not face some of the pressures

---

[1] See https://khn.org/news/public-health-officials-are-quitting-or-getting-fired-amid-pandemic (accessed December 5, 2022).

faced by leaders in government agencies, and should be "willing to lean forward and push to make sure we are highlighting and promoting science and transparency."

Marc Gourevitch from New York University Langone Health offered reflections on academia's role in responding to the pandemic and to racial injustice. With regard to the state of the science and evidence, he listed several examples of areas where the evidence is already available to inform action and policy, such as approaches to reversing chronic disinvestment in Black and Brown communities. In addition to implementing known evidence, truth telling and narrative shifting also are needed to help inform public attitudes and health-related policy, Gourevitch added. He described, as an example, the findings over the past decade about how obesity affected military readiness, and how messaging about those findings was persuasive to a broader range of decision makers (Gollust et al., 2013). What is needed, he added, is a research and action agenda on how to inform the public and decision makers about what produces health that "infuses all of our work and language."

In her remarks, Sheri Johnson from the University of Wisconsin–Madison School of Medicine and Public Health called for addressing the conflation of race and racism in teaching and scholarship and the erroneous use of race, instead of racism, as the explanatory factor for health disparities (Hardeman and Karbeah, 2020). "Unfortunately, in academia" Johnson stated, "we still have an imbalance of how we understand race as a social construct, [how] we teach about it, how we craft the questions that we ask in our scholarship," and academics must face these issues in a comprehensive and direct way, "not as an extracurricular pursuit." Research indicates, added Johnson, that members of the general public as well as medical students and residents have erroneous beliefs that there are biological differences between Blacks and Whites, and these beliefs influence decisions made by public health and health care practitioners. The recognition that racism is an organized and hierarchic social system "based on an ideology of inferiority" strips racism of the power it has to influence the allocation of societal resources, Johnson stated. The recent executive order and related memo from the U.S. Office of Management and Budget that question the use of critical race theory in academia and other organizations makes these reflections timely, Johnson added. Critical race theory is a framework that has been around since the 1980s to examine society, culture, and the intersections with race "pervasive across all aspects of society including housing, employment, education, public health, the law, and it explicitly probes racism's influence on both outcomes and processes." The work of applying these concepts is not aiming to demonize some groups compared to others, Johnson stated, but to serve as a framework for telling the truth about the historical context in which some groups received opportunities and advantages denied to other groups. These truths are the real drivers of differences in health and health outcomes, including the disproportionate burden of COVID-19 in communities of color.

Johnson shared a specific example for how the medical school curriculum reinforces false assumptions about race, describing one university's analysis of medical school lectures, which identified 102 slides that mentioned race. Only 4 percent acknowledged social determinants of racialized disease disparities, compared to 58 percent that implied biological difference (Tsai et al., 2016). Johnson underscored Gourevitch's observation about the need for new narrative framing: the field needs new narratives that decouple race and racism and integrate into teaching and scholarship a fundamental acknowledgment of the societal structures that drive differences in health and health outcomes. Hughes asked if universities have the necessary resources and tools to integrate this information into their curricula and teaching. Johnson replied that the field is still in the early stages of comprehensively interrogating and overhauling curricula and scholarship, and that some approaches, like teaching about cultural humility and implicit bias, are easier to implement than others.

Sharfstein spoke about integrating trauma-informed practices in the curriculum and classroom experience and thinking about the current moment as an opportunity to teach more about responding to crisis, and to do so in a broad-based way, connecting to other disciplines and sectors. It is one thing, said Sharfstein, to conduct epidemiologic work quantifying the pandemic's impact on Black and Latino communities. It is a different matter to be able to respond to these questions of the specific interventions needed, for instance, in the transportation sector or with regard to low-wage jobs. What is the role of public health in these areas? Sharfstein added that leaders in academia need to think of public health as a field that becomes activated in crisis.

Little things, began Ziad Obermeyer from the University of California, Berkeley, can matter a whole lot, and a small, technical issue can put in motion a series of larger actions that can have enormous negative consequences. Obermeyer said that researchers use health care costs to measure health care needs, but recent research he and colleagues conducted showed how an algorithm based on that assumption and used by many health systems around the United States was found to be facilitating "large-scale racial disparities."[2] The algorithms predict how much a patient's care will cost and allocate extra resources for help (e.g., home visits from a nurse practitioner to manage medications), to people who are projected to cost a lot. That means that when people who need health

---

[2] Obermeyer and colleagues published the Algorithmic Bias Playbook, based on their research findings, in June 2021. See https://www.chicagobooth.edu/research/center-for-applied-artificial-intelligence/research/algorithmic-bias/playbook (accessed December 20, 2022).

care do not get health care, they "cost" less (as measured by medical claims) than people who have access to health care. When Obermeyer and his colleagues studied this issue, they learned that this algorithm builds in inequities toward populations of color, those with lower incomes, rural populations, and anyone who lacks adequate health care access or who "is treated differently when they get access to [the] health care system." Obermeyer and colleagues worked with the company that develops the software to change the algorithm to remove the built-in inequity.[3] A similar bias, Obermeyer noted, is built into some government policies. For example, the 2020 Coronavirus Aid, Relief, and Economic Security (CARES) Act included a provision that allocated funding based on an algorithm formulated on the basis of past revenue, which built in racial biases similar to those described above. Because the field does not always have appropriate measures to identify who needs help, there are often no mechanisms or incentives to distribute resources equitably.

Hughes asked how difficult it is to identify alternate measures that do not deepen inequity. Obermeyer said that although the main measure (cost) is available from claims data and other data sets, there is a wealth of additional measures in those data sets that may be more reflective of patient needs, and there also are national data sets that can be used (e.g., blood pressure data that is available from a survey program that gathers the data in people's homes). The data are available, and researchers and practitioners need to understand that these data are valuable both for achieving equitable outcomes and for ensuring effectiveness.

Shreya Kangovi from the University of Pennsylvania shared her reflections on society's and the discipline's inadequate acknowledgment of the current state of inequitable conditions and resulting health disparities. "We are in denial," Kangovi said, and there is evidence that indicates health inequity is a psychological disease that affects the privileged but with symptoms found in the disadvantaged, she noted. Researchers and practitioners study, pathologize, and aim to "improve" people's hemoglobin A1Cs and other measures, but those "experts" need to understand the root cause, which is their own "perverse psychology of the privileged" that manifests itself in inequities. Kangovi added that the field needs to build an implementation science to further critical race theory by partnering with people who experience disadvantage. Community health workers (CHWs), for example, share life experience with the people they serve, Kangovi stated, and the emerging model for the work of CHWs is built on an empowerment framework (Rifkin, 2003). CHWs, Kangovi stated, should not be viewed as a means to the health care system's own targets. Accordingly, health system leaders ought not to say "use" or "get them to" when referring to the roles and contributions of CHWs, but rather, to

---

[3] See https://science.sciencemag.org/content/366/6464/447 (accessed December 5, 2022).

reflect a model of true partnership analogous to how a CHW would ask a community member "what do you think you need?" Such a shift in framing and mindset reflects a transfer of power and control.

Johnson asked Kangovi to reflect on how science is placed on a pedestal, seen as never being wrong or needing to self-correct. Kangovi stated that it is important to first define what is meant by science. If this is about the essence of science as truth telling, as asserted by Hughes, that is indisputable, but the culture of science—its elitism, the blind spots when science is only done by one kind of person—that is problematic. Kangovi stated that the field needs more participatory science or people science.[4] Sharfstein asked Kangovi what she thought about COVID-19 vaccine uptake in the context of the American public's thinking about it. A top-down science way of doing things will not work, and a public relations campaign may not work, she responded. It is necessary to employ an empowerment framework rather than a target-oriented one to engage communities in the implementation of a COVID-19 vaccine.

Sandro Galea from the Boston University School of Public Health outlined what he called three distinct traumas that the nation is experiencing—COVID-19, economics, and the "reckoning with centuries of structural racism"—and these traumas call for strategies for the academic enterprise to deal with them. Galea underscored other speakers' comments calling on academia to speak the truth, to bear witness, and to serve as a moral compass. However, simple and quick solutions will not adequately respond to the traumas that the nation is facing, but academia needs to act on all three planes, Galea stated, specifically to:

1. articulate academia's role in generating the science and evidence to move society forward;
2. rethink the economics of academia, which previously may have allowed (some) academics to feel separate from macroeconomic forces, with secure livelihoods, and to consider who gets to have those roles and benefits; and
3. reckon with centuries of racism, bringing what has long been known to greater public attention.

This calls on academia to look inward and outward to guide how it responds when people are marginalized; how it brings a "stabilizing constructive voice to conversations" both to react to urgent short-term questions and to long-term considerations, such as what is being learned

---

[4] *Participatory science* is sometimes used interchangeably with *citizen science*, referring to engaging a broader range of people in conducting research. See, for example, the discussion in the National Academies report *Learning Through Citizen Science: Enhancing Opportunities by Design* (NASEM, 2018).

and what can be done better in response to COVID-19 and racism. Galea asserted that it is the job of academia to contribute the ideas toward building a better world. Sharfstein added that there are flaws to the academic model, even as society can benefit from its positions and advocacy, and invited others to weigh in about flaws and opportunities.

Reflecting on the then impending election, Kangovi remarked that there is a need to act to help get out the vote. Sharfstein mentioned Vot-ER as one effort in health care to register people to vote.[5] Galea added that voter registration is part of educating Americans about the core responsibilities of a citizen—the nonpartisan notion of civic participation not just in the world of ideas but the in world of action—to vote. Johnson commented on ongoing work to develop measures of civic engagement that are comprehensive and include attention to structural factors, such as the number of election polling stations, voter suppression efforts, and "looking at effects on overall health and differences in health by group," and ultimately making these drivers structural and normative.

DISCUSSION WITH AUDIENCE INPUT

Sharfstein relayed an audience question about recruiting, engaging, and supporting students, especially students from disadvantaged backgrounds, at a time when learning is largely virtual, and students may face many logistical, economic, and public health issues. Sharfstein shared an example about his school's program that has redesigned course offerings.[6] The school additionally provides full scholarships for public health training for 50 people who are working in other sectors to respond to public health challenges, and who may not otherwise be able to receive formal public health training.

A viewer asked if people in the field could put the science that calls for physical distancing in context for people for whom this behavior is impossible because of their living and work circumstances. Johnson spoke about existing solutions for responding to inequities—the direct evidence, or evidence that can be extrapolated, supporting implementation of guaranteed income and increases in Supplemental Nutrition Assistance Program food assistance, the earned income tax credit, and the Great Smoky Mountain Study (Costello et al., 2016). "These are some of the strategies we know can respond to the inequities in society," Gourevitch said. Some of these solutions, such as the economic interventions that could take the pressure off lower-income families, Gourevitch noted, are stuck in con-

---

[5] See https://vot-er.org (accessed December 28, 2020).

[6] See the Bloomberg American Health Initiative at Johns Hopkins University at https://americanhealth.jhu.edu (accessed December 18, 2022).

gressional gridlock. Academia does not think about the political sphere much and avoids entering the political fray. However, he added, this is not about being partisan, but about framing the messaging and narrative to have a greater effect. Obermeyer shared his thinking that the failure to implement testing innovations could have contributed to more targeted stay-at-home policies that could have caused less harm. Hughes reflected on academia's potential role in informing the COVID-19 vaccine rollout to give equitable access to different communities on the ground, but she acknowledged the short time frame available to prepare in this way.

Galea asserted that academia has not had "a trustworthy partner in the public sector." In normal times, the public sector is the best forum to bring society together for problem solving, he noted, but because the sector has not been functioning optimally, the academic inputs have not been weighed by public-sector partners among all inputs and perspectives, and something important has been lost in terms of collaborating to identify solutions. Is there a way for academia to take on some public functions when public-sector entities—such as CDC—are not working effectively, Sharfstein asked. Gourevitch agreed that there is a role for academia to step in and then step back when things improve in the public sector—there are many efforts unfolding to collect COVID-19 data, such as the Johns Hopkins COVID-19 website, and to tell stories about the data being collected. He added that academia has in some ways stepped into the vacuum. It is important to articulate where it can step back again. Sharfstein asked Kangovi to speak about the role of academia to elevate people's lived experiences. The trajectory of inequity in health starts with the psychology of the privileged, she responded, and that shapes the distribution of wealth and power and community, which in turn influences living conditions, behavior, and health. At each step along the way there are possibilities to intervene, and at each point, Kangovi stated, the contributions of people with lived experience should be brought in to inform the interventions.

This discussion raised the issue of the "rules of academia," said Johnson, and ways in which people in academia obtain power through tenure, promotion, and leadership positions. Forms of research that require deep listening and time may not align with the ways in which academics are recognized, Johnson added, and that type of research is needed to inform thinking about the workforce and the nature of academics in public health and population health. In a similar vein, Kangovi commented on the need for leaders in academia to ask themselves what it means "to be a public health student and who can afford to be a student in public health and who gets to do science?" Hughes concluded with a reflection on the fact that schools of public health cannot do it alone; they are dependent on other schools, other sectors, and people with lived experience.

3

Social Sector

The social sector, as reflected in the panel's discussion, encompasses several different dimensions of society. Those include human and social services organizations in the private and public sectors; the faith community in its many manifestations, including congregations and their social activities (e.g., to serve or feed the community) and faith-based nonprofit organizations; and community-based coalitions and partnerships devoted to addressing social, human, and health needs. Milton Little, president of the United Way of Greater Atlanta, introduced the session and the panel, and launched the discussion by asking "What is the most important function of the social sector during two pandemics—COVID-19 and racial injustice?" Key points from the panelists are provided in Box 3-1. Gary Gunderson, vice president for faith–health at Wake Forest Baptist Health and Wake Forest University, remarked that the social sector is often noticed for the minor role it plays as a delivery mechanism for responding to social needs and social risks around the health care sector. However, he asserted, the thing that the sector is best at is social adaptation—the social nature of the creative process by which communities can adapt to predictable and unpredictable threats, from hurricanes to disease outbreaks.

Cathy Baase, board chair of the Michigan Health Improvement Alliance, said it may be too early to have a definitive statement on the role and contribution of the social sector in the pandemic, but she sees the sector's role as a connector, able to convene and unify organizations and facilitate alliances. Susan Dreyfus, president and chief executive officer of the Alliance for Strong Families and Communities, noted that she

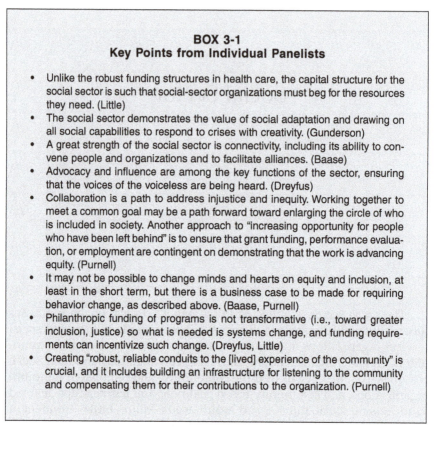

BOX 3-1
Key Points from Individual Panelists

- Unlike the robust funding structures in health care, the capital structure for the social sector is such that social-sector organizations must beg for the resources they need. (Little)
- The social sector demonstrates the value of social adaptation and drawing on all social capabilities to respond to crises with creativity. (Gunderson)
- A great strength of the social sector is connectivity, including its ability to convene people and organizations and to facilitate alliances. (Baase)
- Advocacy and influence are among the key functions of the sector, ensuring that the voices of the voiceless are being heard. (Dreyfus)
- Collaboration is a path to address injustice and inequity. Working together to meet a common goal may be a path forward toward enlarging the circle of who is included in society. Another approach to "increasing opportunity for people who have been left behind" is to ensure that grant funding, performance evaluation, or employment are contingent on demonstrating that the work is advancing equity. (Purnell)
- It may not be possible to change minds and hearts on equity and inclusion, at least in the short term, but there is a business case to be made for requiring behavior change, as described above. (Baase, Purnell)
- Philanthropic funding of programs is not transformative (i.e., toward greater inclusion, justice) so what is needed is systems change, and funding requirements can incentivize such change. (Dreyfus, Little)
- Creating "robust, reliable conduits to the [lived] experience of the community" is crucial, and it includes building an infrastructure for listening to the community and compensating them for their contributions to the organization. (Purnell)

represents America's human service organizations and underscored the sector's influence and advocacy in lifting up the voice of the voiceless in fighting against racial injustices. Jason Purnell from Washington University in St. Louis echoed the commitment to equity but added that community organizations themselves are assessing their own institutional attention to furthering equity and justice. He also acknowledged the extraordinary level of collaboration in the sector. In response to Little's question about the challenges that the sector is facing, Purnell commented on the fiscal and logistical vulnerability—the very existence of organizations is in question as they are forced to operate in new ways in response to the COVID-19 pandemic. Dreyfus added that unrestricted funding is invaluable to the sector, noting that 2020 was the first year that the sector had to begin adapting to the loss of the charitable deduction for tax filers who do not itemize, leading to a decrease in charitable giving. Little shared the findings of a survey of nonprofit organizations in Georgia that showed that most had only 3 months of fiscal reserves on hand before COVID-19 arrived on the scene. He emphasized the funding differences between social-sector organizations that are situated in the health care space and those that are not, with the former receiving Medicaid funding and the latter relying primarily on donations.

Gunderson spoke of the history of the sector, which shows that many social-sector organizations sprang out of a faith-based context. The United States has more than 250,000 religious congregations that people in need turn to, and many of those institutions, perhaps as many as 20 percent of them, are not expected to survive. "How will the durable compassion present in every American community be reconfigured as the nation emerges from this crisis?" Gunderson asked. Underscoring the faith community connections, Little noted that three of the four people who founded the United Way in Denver in 1887 were clergy.

Returning to the question about sustainable funding for the sector, Dreyfus agreed that the field is facing a resource challenge, and asserted that it requires a reassessment of the nation's investments in prisons and other flawed "solutions" that reside at the deep end of the system, instead of investing in vital services, primary care, prevention, and the social determinants of health. What the nation also needs, she added, are opportunities for the health care and social sectors to testify to the same congressional panel advocating for one another—there is a need to combine forces to advocate for "the system that we want to see that produces population health for our neighbors." Gunderson agreed that what is needed are new and more transparent business models (including for health systems, regarding the use of their resources) that allow the social sector to play the roles that it is so well suited to, given its understanding of the social dynamics of people's lives.

Little asked if the social sector will ever be valued for its roles, and Dreyfus responded with a sense of hope. The pandemic, she asserted, has highlighted health inequity and provides an opportunity to consider and address the contexts to people's lives that create inequitable conditions. For example, the evidence about adverse childhood experiences has helped the field understand toxic stress. Health care reform, she noted, focuses on care coordination, prescriptions for food, and other individual-level solutions for a person's needs, but there is a need to address the context to people's lives, which, the field has learned, is shaped by root causes such as systemic racism. Purnell added, however, that it is not enough to present data about health inequity or stir society to a "greater consciousness about systemic racism"; the case must be made that Americans do not have "a viable economy, a viable democracy" if they do not "confront this existential challenge." Baase agreed that the economic case, not merely the altruistic motive, is an important rationale for responding to racial injustice.

Little relayed an audience question on the role of the social sector in shaping or engaging with public narratives (e.g., about the pandemic and strategies to control it), many of which are incorrect, and bridging science and community. Dreyfus spoke about the sector's role in elevating the importance of the stories of human beings. Baase shared that one of the greatest successes of the field is partnership, but division is one of the great societal challenges at the moment. The social sector can bring people together, and it may be easier to accomplish that at the local level and to persuade people to pursue the common good. The current division is troubling, noted Baase, but there are pathways to unity and opportunities to work together.

Faith groups and entities are a great generative factor in communities, Gunderson reflected, but quoted Rosalyn Carter that the first word of faith communities in the public sector should be an apology for their history of stigmatizing behaviors and for being tribal. There is a great need for crossing boundaries and for working across sectors, such as for clergy to get to know and work with their local public health directors, Gunderson said. Being able to draw on the foundational relationships in the community is essential in a crisis such as the current public health emergency. Dreyfus reflected a basic tenet of public-sector work, namely, recognizing the importance of having a two-way relationship. It goes both ways, and social-sector leaders need to recognize that it is the heart of their work to reach out and bridge divides with faith-based entities and others in the community.

Little asked what is needed to build sustainable funding for the social sector. Baase shared that the coalition she is working with seeks to overcome the challenges of scale, sustainability, and coordination. For scale and sustainability, she suggested a funding and financing "utility" (a set of mechanisms) that matches the plan of work. There are other streams beyond philanthropy that can be harnessed for that work, to tie a plan of work from the social sector with a carefully orchestrated range of other funding mechanisms. Examples include drawing on Community Reinvestment Act funding, block grants, deployment and investment of reserve dollars from health systems that have embraced their anchor mission, and so on.

Little asked how the social sector can educate the public and the sectors it works with on the subject of health equity. Purnell shared that as a social scientist, he recognizes that categorizing people is not a "bug" but a feature of human nature. Ultimately, he said, breaking down barriers may be accomplished by bringing people together to work on a common problem. He added that the current crises offer "a real opportunity to rethink who gets included and who is part of this common in-group, and what can we do together."

"I don't think our sector can bring its best self to the table until we have that painful journey," Dreyfus stated, of identifying and responding to implicit bias and the fundamental "rooting" of the human services system in slavery, similar to corrections and other systems. Dreyfus said:

> I think it is really important that before we [try] ... to fix policy and everybody else, I think everyone of us as individuals and as organizations have got to ask ourselves how are we being complicit in this issue.

Baase shared that her organization had made a concerted effort to change its commitments and principles to reflect its values, and made changes in the composition of the board in considering whose voices are represented at all levels of decision making. Purnell underscored the crucial value of "having robust, reliable conduits to the experience of people in the community." Purnell said that this requires a different frame of reference and an openness to listening with intention, as well as building an infrastructure for listening, including a mechanism for compensating community members for their role in informing the work of an organization.

For example, Purnell shared, meetings about gun violence prevention should have someone in the room "who hears gunshots every night, who has had family members and friends shot and killed." Having individuals with lived experience at the decision-making table could accelerate and improve the planning, implementation, and ultimately the outcomes of interventions. Dreyfus spoke about human services organizations, like BakerRipley in Houston, Texas, that use the approach of appreciative inquiry to ascertain if a funder's request will meet the community's needs,[1] and when they hear residents say that that is not what is needed or desired, then the organization communicates that information to the funder. Little added that engaging in this manner ensures that the lived experience of communities is transmitted back to funders.

Gunderson shared how his hospital in Winston-Salem, North Carolina, has a great deal of data and was using it to prioritize its activities in the community. The hospital's neighbors had been conducting asset mapping and other work, and recently the hospital leadership met with community leaders to hear about the community's needs. The hospital had assumed that the "ask" would be for clinical resources, such as a clinic or a mobile van, but

> the presenting challenge was living in a food desert. They knew how to grow tomatoes. They did not need us to bring in a box of tomatoes, but at one point they said, "Where are you purchasing the food for your kitchen?"

---

[1] See https://appreciativeinquiry.champlain.edu/wp-content/uploads/2017/09/The-Gift-of-New-Eyes-Reflecting-on-30-Years-of-Appreciative-Inquiry-in-Organizational-Life.pdf (accessed December 5, 2022).

Gunderson said the community was asking the hospital to provide access to its market as a commercial purchaser, and thereby help the community feed itself. Tracing one of the fault lines in the health care delivery sector, Gunderson noted that health sector leaders who work to improve population health and who interact with the community or faith-based organizations "are not in the revenue cycle." They are not involved in procurement or business decisions, and it is important that they learn to bring internal colleagues in dialogue with community partners and other organizations. There are professionals in the medical industry, he added, who do not see how they can become "a part of the emergence of healthier communities."

Little raised another audience question. How do organizations help leaders and people push past the "I am not a racist" mentality and toward conducting self-inventory? Dreyfus responded that performance is a compelling argument—that organizations are high performing only if they get the best out of their workforce, including the greatest diversity. This requires leadership that is willing to be vulnerable and to be alert to the need to start the journey, and it requires behavior and action. Regarding diversity, Gunderson remarked that "if none of your friends are embarrassed by any of your friends, you are probably not diverse enough. The diversity may be political or faith or racial." Leaders can review their schedule and see who they have had lunch with or met with or listened to, as well as who they quote or "hang out with." Moreover, Gunderson added, "How do we listen to the people who are on the lower paid ranks of our organizations?" Purnell added, quoting Dr. Martin Luther King, Jr., that the law "cannot make a man love me, but it can stop him from lynching me" to assert that although the heart and mind may not be changed, those outcomes are secondary. What matters, Purnell said, is whether or not grant funding, performance evaluation, or employment are contingent on demonstrating that the work is advancing equity and "increasing opportunity for people who have been left out."

Little noted that the philanthropic community faces similar questions about whether it is hindering the fight for equity and diversity in not only the sector, but in the community. Baase echoed Purnell's earlier remarks, noting that she has come to recognize that not everyone values equity, and that instead of waiting for people to change their minds, leaders and organizations need to "build a pathway based upon value and outcomes and the economic case of this to many different parties." Changing consciousness is important, but the field cannot wait for it.

Dreyfus answered Little by underscoring the importance of moving from program thinking to systems change thinking. He reflected on a sense of frustration that a considerable segment of philanthropy remains focused on plans and services instead of affecting systemic change. Dreyfus stated that her organization will no longer accept grants if there is not a policy interface to them. Systems change happens when "regulatory and fiscal mechanisms are aligned to the very practice and policy we believe in," and it is insufficient to focus only at the practice level. Both philanthropy and public sector funders need to expect and fund for systems change, and grantees need the space to work across the continuum and toward systems change. Little shared that he is engaged with launching a racial equity and healing fund. A common question he faces is "What kind of programs are you going to support?" He said he emphasizes that "we have equity challenges in the United States not because there are not enough programs." Echoing Dreyfus' observations, he noted that there are foundational issues,

> groundwater stuff, that we have to be able to cure in order to solve the disparities that are common across criminal justice, housing, health, you name it. And I think it is about systems change.

Gunderson commented that "as long as the social sector is funded in terms of categorical problems that we are considered relevant to, we will never get paid for systems change." He called on the sector to stop being a part of that pathology. Instead, he asserted, the sector should borrow and wield the intellectual tools—such as David Cooperrider's "appreciative inquiry," asset mapping, Arvind Singhal's work on "positive deviance," and insights from the "Leading Causes of Life" Network—to transform itself toward greater intellectual diversity and the crossing of boundaries.

In his closing comments Purnell shared that he feels a sense of hope about the possibility for the sector to move forward strategically, and he underscored earlier comments about the need for the philanthropic funding of system change, not merely of individual organizations or programs. Dreyfus said that it is time to stop talking about health care reform as technical change (e.g., care coordination) and turn to facilitating adaptive change and transforming human services from the inside out to improve population health. "We need to see each other's humanity and lean in with love," she added. Baase spoke about the need for capacity, including the need to fund capacity building in order to achieve systems change, and the need to bring along the next generation of sector leaders.

4

The Health Care Response

Sanne Magnan from the HealthPartners Institute welcomed and introduced the panel on the health care response to the pandemic and the movement for racial justice. She asked panelists Philip Alberti from the Association of American Medical Colleges (AAMC), Dawn Alley from the Centers for Medicare & Medicaid Services (CMS), Kirsten Bibbins-Domingo from the University of California, San Francisco (UCSF), Von Nguyen from the Blue Cross and Blue Shield of North Carolina, and Stella Whitney-West from NorthPoint Health and Wellness to share their thoughts about changes that are needed organizationally, in the community, and in the field and system-wide. Key points from the panelists are provided in Box 4-1.

Alberti shared a story about partnerships. Recently, AAMC gave an award for outstanding community engagement to the Rush College of Medicine in Chicago. Medical students in the service learning program had been working in the city shelter system, which is part of a large partnership that includes health care, government public health, community organizations, and others. The students expressed concern about how heavily the congregate and the partnership sprang into action to administer tests, respond to outbreaks, and ensure continuity of care. Because of all of the planning and collaboration, the entire shelter system in Chicago sustained only two COVID-19 deaths, Alberti noted. According to program leaders, the partnership accomplished more in 5 months than it did in the 20 years prior—the new normal of COVID-19 is a committed partnering and investing in partnership, with COVID-19 acting as a catalyst that calls on an established partnership to be nimble and agile.

BOX 4-1
Key Points from Individual Panelists

- Patient and community engagement as factors in health care delivery system planning and service delivery range from Centers for Medicare & Medicaid Services measures of patient experience to the requirement that federally qualified health centers have at least 51 percent of their boards comprised of patients, to partnerships with community organizations. (Alberti, Alley, Bibbins-Domingo, Whitney-West)
- The pandemic has created an opportunity to broaden use of telehealth, but the greater accessibility for some comes with hurdles for others who may lack the Internet connectivity or technology to link with providers. Organizations need to respond to emerging inequitable conditions. (Bibbins-Domingo)
- Community hubs, such as those situated in libraries, can offer sites for community residents to access telehealth services. (Whitney-West)
- The health system's embrace of its mission as an anchor—realigning procurement, hiring, and other dimensions—is an important perspective that extends to its COVID-19 response. (Bibbins-Domingo)

Nguyen shared how his organization started its own exploration of its role in advancing equity. His system recognized the large policy questions raised by the 2020 protests against racial injustice. The system recognized that it is not a primary actor on many of the aspects, but it still had an opportunity to participate as part of a larger partnership, as well as through structural changes. Nguyen remarked that the system recognized that network adequacy is one approach to help advance equity. Network adequacy, he explained, refers to the requirement that health care plans have providers in every zip code to ensure adequate coverage for its insurance policies. In a rural area, that provider could be 20 miles away, and although that may technically meet the definition, it is not really adequate and is inconsistent with the goal of advancing equity.

Alley remarked that the system is generally better at measuring issues related to cost and quality than those related to access, and the agency is grappling with how to measure access effectively. She acknowledged that health plans may not be enthusiastic about having network adequacy requirements increased, but she appreciates that some plans are engaging around those issues in a meaningful way.

Bibbins-Domingo said that organizations need to think internally about what they are uniquely poised to do. UCSF launched health equity councils at both of its hospitals and reviewed ways to integrate equity principles into all of its data collection on quality and safety and patient experience. Although the report *Unequal Treatment: Confronting Racial and*

Ethnic Disparities in Health Care (IOM, 2003) was released almost 20 years ago, a lot of these issues, even the measures, are not universally embraced. The pandemic has affected hospital finances, but the university has been involved in robust community partnerships, working effectively with public health to drive improvement.

Alberti asked if there is any movement to get community and patient input into what makes a network adequate. Nguyen shared that his organization is in the early stages of working on this issue. He noted that there is work to be done on the system definition of what is technically adequate on paper versus what network adequacy means from the members' or patients' standpoint.

Alley shared that on the Medicare program side there are a number of measures of patient experience that deal with trust, communication, availability, and timeliness of care. With regard to value-based payment in Medicare, the problem is likely to be people getting too much care or the wrong types of care (e.g., unnecessary testing, lack of coordinated care, multiple care coordinators). In the Medicaid context, Alley noted, the issue is people not getting care at all, and there also are difficulties in facilitating access to care in rural settings.

Stella Whitney-West, whose organization is a federally qualified health center (FQHC), shared aspects of her health center's work that ground it in the community and underscore its relationship with community members. Whitney-West said that more than 70 percent of her health center's staff is from the community, and 51 percent of the board is comprised of patients of the health center (a requirement for FQHCs). As part of the response to racial injustice, the health center focused on the emotional well-being of staff, who are drawn from the community and are primarily people of color. For example, the health center organized a protest march around the neighborhood, led by staff who are African drummers, and the community responded. This idea emerged from daily staff huddles that are not clinically focused, but are rather centered on having a "mindful moment" in addition to receiving COVID-19 updates and building team togetherness at the start of each day.

Alley shared her perspective about responding to the twin crises unfolding in the context of massive transformation occurring as the U.S. health system moves to value-based payments. Data and flexibility are needed for value-based care to be successful. What Alley noticed in the first months of the pandemic is that the providers who had been investing in transforming care "were better poised to be nimble and respond to this changing dynamic, ramp up telehealth, engage care teams, and track patients—all the things you really needed to be able to do to deliver effective care." She shared how the U.S. Department of Health and Human Services is focusing on maternal morbidity and mortality both in general and in the context of issues that have emerged during COVID-19. Telehealth has emerged as a potential benefit of the new environment—it makes care more accessible for some patients, but there are also barriers. There is an opportunity created by the pandemic to do things that are more patient centered and accessible, but there is also a risk of perpetuating or exacerbating disparities if people lack the technology or Internet access, Alley noted.

Regarding technology access, Bibbins-Domingo commented on the communication challenges presented by language and cultural differences, and the ongoing efforts to find solutions. It is essential to recognize, she noted, that telehealth services are here to stay, but there are equity issues that need to be resolved. Nguyen shared that the Blue Cross Blue Shield of North Carolina saw a 7,000 percent increase in telehealth use. Telehealth services provide a great solution for an essential worker needing to take a day off, needing parking—barriers that are hard to overcome—but it can create inequities. For example, although telehealth has worked well for behavioral health care, there are some challenges, such as creating a therapeutic environment when people are home and surrounded by their children, or if circumstances cause them to be outside their home, such as shopping in a grocery store. It will be crucial, Nguyen noted, that systems ensure that telehealth can be a conduit for the same high-quality care that a patient would expect from an in-person visit.

Whitney-West spoke about her FQHC's focus on providing care to patients regardless of ability to pay, but they also offer the services of the health center's eligibility support staff to enable patients who may be unaware of their eligibility status to access care in other settings. To address patients' challenges with Internet access, technology, and even data plan constraints, the health center replicated an idea it had learned about and created telehealth hubs around the community to help ensure access for patients. Hennepin County has a network of libraries and community locations where the health center established private offices where people could go to for telehealth visits, and community health workers are available to assist as needed.

Alberti commented on how this story clearly illustrated the difference between having an insurance card and actually having access to health care. He then shared a personal anecdote from someone who had been a skeptic about the federal government's ability to afford universal access. The person had an epiphany that if the federal government can manage to fund a $1 trillion program (the COVID-19 stimulus), the lack of universal health coverage in the United States is not about cost but reflects societal choices. Clearly, COVID-19 has brought into high relief, in addition to injustice and inequity, "the fact that it is possible to make different choices when a crisis hits. The question for the nation to ask itself is how that momentum can be maintained to rethink what is possible."

Bibbins-Domingo reflected on Alberti's comment about the true meaning of access and shared that UCSF took its COVID-19 testing directly into the community rather than wait for people to come to it. Although the Latino community makes up about 15 percent of the population in San Francisco, it accounts for more than 50 percent of the COVID-19 cases, and the health system learned much by partnering with community organizations to set up neighborhood-based testing sites. UCSF learned how to deal with misinformation about payment, care, and what it would mean for job security, immigration status, and being considered a public charge. She added that it was the community-based organizations who did all of the follow up, linking people to resources and services they needed from food to even housing if someone needed to quarantine away from their household. Magnan noted that one audience question touched on misinformation. Bibbins-Domingo shared that in marginalized communities, COVID-19, injustice, and economic instability interact to contribute to misinformation, and marginalization feeds misinformation.

Nguyen said that his health plan, with leadership from the chief executive officer, found it critical to reinforce the messages coming from the North Carolina Department of Health about wearing masks and handwashing. Health systems, working through the providers, are often trusted actors in the community, which positions them to play an important role in being trusted communicators. The health plan worked with health systems and the business community in the state to disseminate trusted information coming from the Department of Health. That public–private partnership played an important role. Bibbins-Domingo shared how her health system worked with community-based organizations to communicate to the community in different languages, including Cantonese, Spanish, and Vietnamese, and respond to the real hunger for information it noticed in the community. Before COVID-19, Bibbins-Domingo added, the health system had made the commitment to embrace its role as an anchor institution and therefore realign its procurement and hiring to be an economic player in the local community. That is an important perspective that the organization brings to its COVID-19 response as well.

Magnan asked Alley if the Medicare policy team has considered paying for outcomes and disparity reduction, under the assumption that reimbursement of funding would drive change and better outcomes more quickly than many other methods. Alley said yes and noted that there is an upcoming meeting of a National Quality Forum (NQF) technical panel that will consider adjustments for social risk.[1] CMS is focused on balancing the need to establish incentives to close the equity gaps in providing

---

[1] For a definition of social risk, see NASEM (2017): "Social risk factors capture how social relationships and contexts influence the health care outcomes of Medicare beneficiaries."

high-quality care to everyone, particularly to those who need it most and ensuring high quality of care while avoiding potentially penalizing safety net providers. The agency is also considering different ways to collect social risk information, such as the Area Deprivation Index, which has been used in the Maryland cost of care model.

Health inequities related to COVID-19 have drawn attention to the dual-eligible population and population with end-stage renal disease as two very vulnerable groups. CMS is also focusing on quality measurement and data standardization in the context of the accountable health communities model, and it is collecting data on a large scale on health-related social needs such as housing instability and food insecurity. As a general insight, Alley shared that it is easier to measure processes than outcomes, and CMS aims to gather more information about what works and how to measure it.

Alberti said that he is a co-chair of the NQF disparity standing committee, and that the committee has been overseeing a trial period of social risk adjustment for the past several years. That work is being concluded, and a subsequent expert panel will be reconvened soon. System leaders fear using social risk adjustment and having that mask inequity or allow for a lower standard of care, Alberti noted, but the data can be stratified. The greater challenge is that social risk data do not inform risk adjustment in a valid way. One approach is to try to adjust for Black race versus everybody else, but being Black is not a risk factor and "there's no intervention for Black race—it's not even a real thing," he added. "Racism is the risk factor." The other approach is to adjust for dual eligibility. Evidence indicates that dual-eligible patients receive poor quality of care, and that is related to the social determinants of health and individual social risks that the patient experiences in the clinical encounter, Alberti stated. What is needed in the future, he said, is a

> national, standardized social risk data collection system that has a strategy and a plan, and that allows all of our sectors to avail ourselves of that information, so it allows the clinician to provide better care. It allows public health departments to craft better interventions. It allows CMS to make smarter adjustments based on the mechanisms of injustice that create inequities, beside readmission [metrics].

Bibbins-Domingo said that the metrics available for risk adjustment, despite their limitations, are still useful if health systems like hers are given incentives not just for meeting targets (e.g., lowering hypertension), but for closing the gaps. Alberti noted that "tracking the gaps is not the same as measuring equity" unless a metric exists that can capture whether patients of any background feel they receive the same equitable opportunity for high-quality health care as "a White, cisgender, heterosexual, Judeo-Christian, rich man."

Whitney-West commented that her FQHC is part of the Hennepin County government, which has declared racism a public health crisis. Health care often treats the symptoms but does not address the root cause; therefore, the county government built in metrics and goals, including furthering equity through county contracts and vendors. Looking at housing, benefits, employment, and other factors that help ensure equity in the population, these are all a part of what public- and private-sector organizations can do to address historic racism, such as when the county locked people out of opportunity through policies such as redlining and Whites-only housing covenants.

Magnan relayed an audience question about the fact that community health centers have a legal requirement to have a majority of their boards comprised of patients, and whether this could be made into a requirement for other clinical care organizations. Whitney-West said that patients on the governing board bring their perspectives and tools to the table—they are messengers and trusted sources with the community. Her message to other health care organizations is that they are missing an opportunity if they do not find ways to include their constituents, community, or patients in their organization in a meaningful way. Alberti said that there are organizations that have several boards—Massachusetts General Hospital is one that has four boards—for research, education, clinical care, and community. There are many examples of perfunctory, box-checking engagement, but there also is momentum to incorporate patient and community voice in ways that "share power and lead to real change."

Bibbins-Domingo shared that her organization launched a patient community advisory board related to COVID-19 to both inform research related to COVID-19 as well as for community input on UCSF COVID-19 testing projects. She added that the advisory board exemplifies bidirectional communication and learning. A number of Center for Medicare & Medicaid Innovation models, stated Alley, include requirements for some type of community input or engagement, which may offer an opportunity to build in this important input. On a related note, Alley mentioned a call for feedback from Johns Hopkins University on ways to develop measures of the health of the community surrounding the hospital as an indicator of hospital quality.

Magnan noted that an audience member asked about the implications for health care of the call in the business community to diversify boards. Alberti clarified that IBM Watson Health's hospital rankings initiative asked Johns Hopkins to develop a metric that attempts to capture a hospital's contribution to community health and equity, but it also reflects on institutional culture, climate, gender equity, and so forth. The Lown Institute has a new metrics set that aims to assess health care organization performance on the organization's civic leadership, the value of care it provides, and patient outcomes.[2] There are, he added, some formal community benefit forms that attempt to capture some of the free care as well as aspects of community health improvement activity by hospitals. The challenge, Alberti noted, is identifying a national metric that captures the institution's effort at community health improvement and whether it is responsive to the identified needs of the local community.

Magnan asked a final audience question about mental health services in the context of the pandemic. Nguyen said that his health system views this through three different lenses: (1) supporting employees by helping them manage behavioral health challenges; (2) providing access to mental and behavioral health care via telehealth for substance use disorder, depression secondary to COVID-19, and serious mental illness; and (3) in the community, engaging especially through their foundation in strategies to respond to social isolation and loneliness. Whitney-West noted that her health center provides school-based services, too, and a component of that is mental health. She also reflected on the fact that mental and behavioral health has been devalued in the United States, and the most striking examples occur in the context of police brutality, such as the cases where law enforcement arrives on the scene and community members experiencing a mental health crisis get injured or killed.

Alley quoted James Baldwin in that "not everything that is faced can be changed, but nothing can be changed until it is faced." Alley said "we're facing a lot of things right now, but we need to be able to continue to see them, and the language of health care is data and incentives and reimbursements, so we need to figure out how to take this conversation and really face" the need for change in the context of issues such as data and payment. Alberti asked how the data and the opportunities discussed can be leveraged to "position health care [entities] as a partner in developing a health agenda, and not just a health care agenda." Nguyen added that beyond the data, what is needed is understanding the role of culture. Magnan emphasized the importance of feeling discomfort about the role of institutions and the need for leaders such as those on the panel to dig deeper. Whitney-West closed by remarking that the current crisis is one that the nation has been in for decades, and Americans have just become numb to it.

---

[2] See https://lowninstitute.org/press-release-can-2020-push-hospitals-from-good-to-great (accessed December 18, 2022).

5

Public Health

John Auerbach of Trust for America's Health introduced the conversation with a question about how public health is navigating this challenging time of both the pandemic and the movement against racial injustice. Key points from the panelists are provided in Box 5-1.

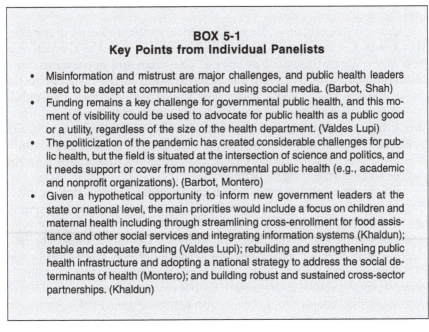

BOX 5-1
Key Points from Individual Panelists

- Misinformation and mistrust are major challenges, and public health leaders need to be adept at communication and using social media. (Barbot, Shah)
- Funding remains a key challenge for governmental public health, and this moment of visibility could be used to advocate for public health as a public good or a utility, regardless of the size of the health department. (Valdes Lupi)
- The politicization of the pandemic has created considerable challenges for public health, but the field is situated at the intersection of science and politics, and it needs support or cover from nongovernmental public health (e.g., academic and nonprofit organizations). (Barbot, Montero)
- Given a hypothetical opportunity to inform new government leaders at the state or national level, the main priorities would include a focus on children and maternal health including through streamlining cross-enrollment for food assistance and other social services and integrating information systems (Khaldun); stable and adequate funding (Valdes Lupi); rebuilding and strengthening public health infrastructure and adopting a national strategy to address the social determinants of health (Montero); and building robust and sustained cross-sector partnerships. (Khaldun)

Joneigh Khaldun, chief medical officer of the Michigan Department of Health, said that this is a moment of pride for public health. Her state health department began its planning for COVID-19 in January. Oxiris Barbot, former health commissioner of New York City, said that people need to acknowledge that this is a mixed time for public health in that the disconnect among federal, state, and local response to the pandemic has been a challenge, but it has also been an opportunity because it is kind of a Super Bowl for public health, allowing the field to demonstrate the deep bench that it has. Although it is a difficult time (i.e., protecting the health of the community), it is a good time for the field to distinguish itself from health care (i.e., providing clinical care to individuals). Monica Valdes Lupi, senior program officer at The Kresge Foundation and former Boston public health commissioner, agreed that this is a time of both challenges and opportunity for public health.

José Montero, director of the Center for State, Territorial, Local, and Tribal Support at the Centers for Disease Control and Prevention (CDC), said that one of the challenges in the pandemic response has been the evolving science, but he added that the system's capacity to respond has been impressive. He noted that the preparations for a pandemic did not just begin with the emergence of COVID-19, but that planning had been taking place for years—he worked on pandemic response planning years ago as a state health official. The pandemic has also highlighted the need for collaboration and integration with health care, and it has also had inequitable effects on the population, with some groups becoming sick and dying at higher rates.

Umair Shah, executive director and local health authority of the Harris County Department of Public Health, agreed with the characterization of the current moment as both a "challenge and opportunity," but also commented on the often politicized nature of the response to the pandemic. He talked about addressing the invisibility crisis that public health faces using three Vs: raise visibility, which brings value, which in turn brings validation in the form of prohealth policies and/or prohealth resources. Shah said that he just never thought that it would be a fourth V—virus—that would actually raise the profile of public health to the degree that it has during COVID-19.

Auerbach asked the panel about the key lessons from this moment. Barbot commented that risk communication has been critical in responding to the pandemic, and she spoke about how in the response in New York City early, frequent, clear, and consistent communication to residents was critical, as were openness about what was known and areas of unknowns or uncertainty. Having messaging reinforced by leaders in other sectors is similarly important. Barbot expressed concern about how young people considering public health careers regard the targeting and scapegoating of public health leaders in the pandemic. She said that she would want young people to recognize the value of public service and of bringing science to the everyday lives of Americans. That is a value that must be protected, she added. Khaldun spoke about the importance of equipping public health professionals, epidemiologists, and scientists with the skills to communicate effectively with leaders in other sectors, including political leaders, and with the ability to translate scientific information in a clear and relevant way.

Montero concurred with Khaldun's comment about communication and added that being able to communicate uncertainty is crucial. Better transmission and translation of data to the public is important, as the public now has more access to certain facts and figures on their phones than ever before. It has been an interesting dichotomy in working with the public that is hungry for information about where people are sick while at the same time "many of them don't want to tell us when they were sick or who they were with when we are asking them to do contact tracing."

Valdes Lupi said that community engagement is an important element of the larger communication effort. For example, "we will need to lean on community partners to roll out a vaccination program." In some jurisdictions, like Boston, there is a high uptake of immunizations, but in some areas, the level of trust is lower and influenza vaccine uptake is low. Communicating complicated issues to the public is a challenge, so working with trusted community partners is crucial. Shah summarized some of the communication skills that public health leaders need but may lack, from risk communications to social media to being able to communicate complex topics clearly and in a reassuring, not scary, manner during times of crisis.

Auerbach added that another important lesson is to respond to the available data about the misery and death in populations of color and to work on issues related to promoting equity. There were two audience questions on that theme, Auerbach noted. How can public health, particularly governmental public health, be influenced to prioritize Black and Latino communities and other populations of color who are disproportionately represented among those who are most affected by COVID-19? Second, how does the field address social factors such as living wages, expanding Medicaid coverage, and ensuring that people have affordable quality housing?

Shah answered first that COVID-19 did not start these inequities, although those preexisting inequities have unfortunately been accentuated and worsened by the pandemic across the nation. Public health has a responsibility, just as it did prior to (and well after) the pandemic, to address the structural and social factors that shape health outcomes. For example, Khaldun said, people need to vote, and greater diversity is needed both in public health and in different levels of leadership. It is also necessary to be intentional and systematic about addressing equity. Michigan has an equity impact assessment that the state is implementing, assessing the impact of every policy decision on communities of color, and Khaldun emphasized the importance of having data that has been disaggregated by race and ethnicity.

Barbot spoke about how the New York City Health Department has worked to apply a racial equity lens to change the character of its response, and how it has worked to secure better data to inform its work. However, she noted, public health should not allow itself to be imprisoned by imperfect data. Early in the pandemic, when the agency started to see that Black and Brown New Yorkers were dying at twice the rate of White New Yorkers, the health department sounded the alarm even in the context of incomplete data. Public health needs courageous leaders, and being courageous means being able to make hard decisions in light of imperfect data—which is the definition of public health, Barbot said. She added, "To have more courageous leaders in public health, we need a civil society that supports the value of public health." Public health data should be used, Barbot said, to respond to housing insecurity, food insecurity, and to make it easy for people to follow public health guidance, such as for isolation and quarantine.

Montero spoke about the assets that public health brings to the table in the conversation about the social factors that shape health outcomes. Although public health cannot solve the challenges related to employment, housing, or education, public health has the ability to view health issues and health outcomes in the context of the society and community where life happens. Perhaps public health leaders and workers are not able to change the factors that shape health or the burden of COVID-19, but when public health takes its seat at the tables where those conversations happen, Montero stated, public health has the duty and the ability to raise those issues, and to show how policies in non-health sectors affect health.

Regarding the role of data, Valdes Lupi underscored their importance for policy decisions. Policy and advocacy are highlighting how employment-related issues are contributing to disproportionate COVID-19 burdens in communities of color. Public health leaders understand the value of policies about sick leave benefits, living wages, and stable housing, Valdes Lupi said, and can partner with others to help in addressing these complex issues. An added consideration, noted Valdes Lupi, is the intergenerational effects of these factors on morbidity and trauma for racial and ethnic minority populations. Montero noted that adverse childhood experiences, which affect some populations to a greater degree, are a major issue that public health will need to address through policy and action to lead to "better conditions for children today" that could yield dramatic results for "prevention down the road."

Auerbach agreed with key observations made by the panel and shared a few thoughts, including that categorical funding sometimes makes it difficult to work outside of the disease model, and that the issue of racism can be viewed as controversial in some areas and can be challenging for a public health official to speak about. He shared this to set the stage for a scenario that he presented to panelists. Imagine, he said, a state where a new governor was just elected, and the governor comes in and asks for advice. Khaldun started by sharing the actual advice that she provided to her governor about the need to focus on children and maternal health. The state has focused on expanding Medicaid and finding funding for it, and on streamlining cross-enrollment for food stamps and other social services, by integrating information systems.

Barbot said that in order to measure the effect of policies in different sectors on health outcomes, she would focus on premature mortality. "We know," she said, "that Black, Brown and Indigenous Americans die much earlier than their White counterparts." Valdes Lupi said that she would, as she did in Boston, implement training on antiracism and work to operationalize an equity ethos through equitable procurement policy, such as contracting with community vendors, to invest in local neighborhoods and minority-owned businesses. Administration and finance may not be glamorous activities, but they are critical in rounding out the work of the public health workforce so that resources are allocated to the breadth of key public health issues.

Montero said that he would propose to his hypothetical new governor a 4- or 8-year plan and would focus on the unique geography and other characteristics of the state. Climate change, urbanicity, and other factors may be issues. A state public health leader needs robust capabilities to rely on from data infrastructure to community support, but such a leader also needs flexibility and political support. Shah added that a governor's political antecedents are equally important. What did the governor run on and prioritize, especially related to health? The political naïveté of public health leaders will not serve them well in the face of a lack of political will. Barbot said that "we often talk about the art and science of medicine, but we don't talk about the art and science of public health." The latter, she said, is the ability to present an investment that has long-term gains in a way that makes the short-term gains more apparent. Public health leaders need to be less naïve and more opportunistic in terms of being clear-eyed advocates for their communities, presenting ideas that have the greatest promise for reducing and eliminating racial inequities.

Auerbach thanked panelists, and began fielding additional questions from the audience.

One was, "How do public health leaders combat misinformation about vaccines and about COVID-19?" Shah said that public health leaders need to be active and engaged on social and other media that communities themselves are involved with, but they also need to recognize the potential shortfalls of different media as they utilize them. Barbot shared her experience responding to the 2019 measles outbreak in New York City. In addition to being in front early with "consistent, concise, approachable, accessible information about what the facts are and addressing misinformation head on," she said that engaging trusted community members is essential for sharing messages effectively.

Another audience member asked about the steady decrease in public health funding due to, as Auerbach added, the failure to replenish what was lost in the 2008 recession, along with tens of thousands of public health jobs lost.[1] The pandemic has further decreased government resources at all levels. Montero spoke about the fact that health departments never recovered at the jurisdictional level from the recession, and the pandemic has had an additional effect. Montero spoke about braiding funding (i.e., using separate funding streams in an integrated way to achieve aims shared by different programs), about leveraging resources, and about partnering with other sectors, especially health care. Public health will also need to integrate some of its silos, and that may help. Ultimately, he stated, "We as a society pick and choose what type of government we set, and what type of programs and actions that program, that government is going to implement. We cannot separate one from the other."

Public health is a public good, remarked Valdes Lupi, and the field is no longer invisible; there is a need to take advantage of this moment of visibility to advocate for public health as a public good, like schools, law enforcement, and other services. She added that it has been particularly difficult for smaller jurisdictions to obtain adequate personal protective equipment and resources for setting up mobile testing sites.

An audience member asked, "How should public health grapple with political interference?" Public health, Barbot said, is situated at the intersection of science and politics, and at this particular moment, science is "taking it on the chin." It is important at this time that governmental public health and nongovernmental public health work together,[2] and the latter can support government public health officials that are protecting their communities. Montero said that transparency in science, data, and policy making is a key factor on this. Public health is a participatory

---

[1] See Trust for America's Health reports on public health funding. See https://www.tfah. org/issue-details/public-health-funding (accessed June 23, 2021).

[2] Academia, nonprofit organizations, and public health philanthropy.

decision-making process, and public health needs to recognize that it is not the only messenger and that it needs to work with others to communicate the science. Barbot underscored Montero's observation about transparency, adding that when politics begin to infringe on decision making, a previously high level of transparency will be affected in an indication of the effect of politicization.

Auerbach asked the panelists to turn their attention to a lightning round. The election is over, he said, and the president has been elected. "You get a call from someone who is working on policy, and they are asking you: what's the one thing you would recommend that is the key thing that would advance the health of the population?" he asked.

Khaldun would say to build out a national strategy on COVID-19 and to "rebuild trust in public health and the scientific community." Barbot would call for a "national health equity action plan" that focused on funding public health to target communities that are facing the greatest inequities and that also questions why the United States still has primarily employer-based health insurance in light of the fact that job losses due to COVID-19 have also meant loss of health insurance. Shah would call for ending the devaluation of public health, for supporting and elevating federal agencies like CDC to their previous status, and for ensuring that CDC's work is well coordinated with state and local public health partners. Valdes Lupi would recommend an infusion of resources into public health infrastructure, such as the $4.5 billion that has been recommended by the recent Trust for America's Health report (2020), and she would recommend moving away from the categorical funding of the past. Montero would propose a two-pronged approach: first, rebuild and improve public health infrastructure; second, address core capabilities and functions as part of a national strategy that aims to tackle health issues through addressing the social determinants of health.

Shah said that he would raise the position of governmental public health so that it is no longer subsumed under another agency, but is placed at the highest levels of government, for example, at the federal level as a cabinet-level position or at the state level as a secretary-level position. Khaldun said that she would draw attention to the nation's mental health needs, given the collective trauma that the nation is currently experiencing, its effects on children, and its consequences for generations to come. Also, she added, public health needs strategic partnerships with business, education, health care, and others so that when the next pandemic hits, the sector is ready. Valdes Lupi built on Khaldun's comment by underscoring the importance of building on the strengths and assets of communities and their resilience during this time. Also, the work of public health needs to be trauma informed in order to respond to the trauma and health inequities that communities of color have been experiencing for generations.

Montero concluded by stating that society is experiencing a kind of posttraumatic stress disorder, and that an integrated response will be needed. Moreover, the opioid epidemic is continuing, and the pandemic is uncovering and intensifying other health issues. All of these issues, along with ending the pandemic, are all on the public health sector's long to-do list.

6

Transforming Philanthropy

Phyllis Meadows, senior fellow in health at The Kresge Foundation, welcomed the panel on philanthropy, which was intended to explore the sector's conceptual and practical responses to the pandemic and the movement for racial justice, as well as challenges faced by the field and the prospect of sustained, long-term improvements. Meadows began with brief remarks about the sector's flexibility and responsiveness to grantees during the pandemic. This is a time of social reckoning, she continued, with racial injustice and a history that "demands transformation in philanthropic practice, policy, and investment." There is also economic uncertainty, concerns about American democracy, and a range of other challenges. She introduced the panel: Jacqueline Martinez Garcel, chief executive officer of the Latino Community Foundation; William Buster, vice president of Saint David's Foundation; Marion Standish, vice president for enterprise programs at The California Endowment; Rose Green, senior program officer at the Colorado Health Foundation; and Michelle Larkin, associate executive vice president at the Robert Wood Johnson Foundation. Key points from the panelists are provided in Box 6-1.

Jacqueline Martinez Garcel stated that the current moment has revealed a need for change, particularly to address the legacy of "centuries of racism embedded in our system and policy." Yet, this time also has inspired a sense of hope, she said. One of the challenges is to sustain that hope and the momentum to engage and vote, hold leaders accountable, and demand change to lead to "sustainable public health changes, housing changes, and educational changes." William Buster shared his

---

BOX 6-1
Key Points from Individual Panelists

- To advance racial justice, philanthropic organizations must work internally and externally to change the status quo, which includes a lack of diversity in the field (Buster), a majority of people of color leaving the field in the first 5 years (Green), the devastating role of racism in shaping thinking about philanthropy, and the requirements that philanthropic organizations place on community grantees. (Martinez Garcel)
- The work of philanthropy can unleash community and people power by providing places and opportunities for making connections and planning, providing long-term support, and connecting grantees with the larger ecosystem of data generation and legal assistance. (Green, Martinez Garcel, Standish)
- To support grantees, philanthropic leaders need to share more than just funding. They need to share their knowledge and contacts. (Buster)
- Consider options for longer-term and more sustainable funding models to support not only programs, but also power building and movement building in communities, including program-related investments, impact investing, supervised guarantees, and low-market loans. (Larkin, Martinez Garcel, Standish)

---

own sense of hopefulness in seeing—both in his personal circle and more broadly around the country—that families, communities, and neighborhoods are engaging in dialogue in unprecedented ways. Michelle Larkin commented on the recognition that economic hardships and racial injustice have not just been revealed by the COVID-19 pandemic but have been a reality for many decades. She reflected on how various systems, including philanthropy, have contributed to inequities for people across the country, and this moment is calling for rethinking and transformation.

Marion Standish reflected on the historical context for the current time and emphasized that the truth is finally "being seen and heard on issues and challenges that Black communities, communities of color, and Indigenous communities have been living with for all these years." Rose Green agreed with previous remarks and shared Dr. Martin Luther King, Jr.'s quote about the long arc of the moral universe bending toward justice. "In many ways," she said, "so many of us have become comfortable or apathetic about a system we are all a part of that is an inequitable system built on inequity" and that this is "a revolutionary moment" that provides an opportunity for change.

Meadows asked the panelists to describe how their foundations have begun to pivot in the midst of these challenges. Standish shared that her foundation's major change has been its increased speed in getting resources to affected communities in addition to greater flexibility and more operating funding for grantees. During the pandemic's first month, the foundation made 21 grants amounting to $5 million in new dollars in 72 hours. Martinez Garcel stated that her community foundation's focus is on unleashing the civic power of Latinos in California, and during the pandemic, it has been paying much greater attention to supporting "power builders and movement builders" and finding ways to address needs for "food, transportation, things that were happening with wild-fires, people losing jobs impacted by COVID-19," and other challenges being faced by nonprofit leaders that the foundation supports. Larkin shared that the foundation spent $50 million in humanitarian aid to help families and communities most affected by the "long-term policy failures that we put into place as a nation," leading to needs for "food, housing, and things like rent support," particularly among "communities that have suffered the greatest inequities—communities of color, lower-income workers, and Indigenous communities."

Larkin underscored the earlier remarks about speed and her organization's focus on lessening the burden of reporting and removing burdens in awarding grants to nonprofits that are providing on-the-ground emergency services. Larkin added that as the COVID-19 pandemic is ravaging Black and Indigenous people and communities and other communities of color, the foundation is rising to speak as a national voice "to the public about racial equity in particular and how this is not a political issue; it should not be a partisan issue." The question is, said Larkin,

> How do we as a country rally and move forward to make sure that communities and people, no matter what job they do, where they live, how much money they make, have every opportunity to have a fair and just access and opportunity to health and well-being?

Meadows asked panelists how philanthropic organizations could keep this moment of expansion from contracting back into the old mode of operating. Martinez Garcel shared that it is essential that people in the field recognize that "racism has played a devastating role in how we think about philanthropy" and that "they are part of the problem." Holding a mirror to themselves is crucial, and philanthropic organizations, she asserted, need to trust the people on the ground to do the work and discard reporting requirements. There are also leaders in philanthropy who are concerned about unsupportive boards, but there are ways to bring on board people who "get it" and who will use their abilities to facilitate and support change.

Buster pointed to the webcast window with images of the six speakers and remarked on its racial, ethnic, and gender diversity, but he added that does not reflect how the field looks. "Each of us have agency in our organization, if we have the power to hire and to contract, and it is essential to reassess annually how the field is doing and hold each other accountable."

Standish built on Martinez Garcel and Buster's comments and spoke to both the internal and external aspects of the deliberate work her organization has undertaken to advance racial equity over the past 2 years. The foundation's journey has included examining its use of the language of White supremacy. The internal work has been comprehensive, including reviewing vendors, investing, and grant-making staff. In its externally facing work, the foundation needs to spend more on its partners, Standish noted, asking "How can we spend in a way that gives our partners the room and maneuverability they need to operate effectively?"

Larkin commented that foundations are required by the Internal Revenue Service to pay out no less than 5 percent of their endowment each year. Her foundation, she stated, has focused on spending more than the 5 percent, and investing to support community power. Internally, the organization has focused on reviewing its hiring and contracting, and being explicit in examining "the connection between racism and health and health equity and the inequity that communities of color have suffered and continue to suffer." Echoing Martinez Garcel, Larkin underscored the importance of acknowledging the origins of philanthropic funds, the importance of removing barriers to resources and services that people need, and the "real opportunity to do a better job of listening and understanding how we can work together to create the solutions that we hope to see in our nation."

Green expressed a concern about a likely future contraction after this moment is over. The field needs to "recognize this moment is a long moment." She also said that accountability is a key issue, particularly in some contexts. Privately endowed foundations, small family foundations, and others may not have robust mechanisms or *any* mechanisms for accountability, innovating, changing, or truly moving the work of equity forward, internally and externally. Green shared a recent report from Emerging Practitioners in Philanthropy, of which she is a member. The report *Dissonance & Disconnects* highlighted that a majority of staff of color who have joined philanthropy plan on leaving within the first 5 years "because they don't feel supported [or] welcomed, or they don't feel like they can do the work they want" (EPIP, 2018). Philanthropic organizations "need to think about how to institutionalize the changes so people can feel supported and move up and have influence rather than just being frontline staff."

Meadows asked panelists how they can ensure that the field can be welcoming of diverse newcomers. Buster shared that he invites staff to "bring themselves into the office" and bring "the culture from which they come." How people process things on a cultural level, he noted, informs how they ask questions, make decisions, and move around in their communities. This is an intentional process that can make people uncomfortable because it is challenging the dominant culture, but he added that things do not improve without struggle.

Meadows posed the next question: Have foundations eliminated caps on indirect (i.e., not program) support as a means of support, and will this change continue past COVID-19? Larkin said that her foundation benefited from the work that other philanthropic organizations have done to get at the true cost for grantees, and it has increased indirect support to 20 percent this year and does not intend to reverse that direction, but will continue to reassess whether that is the correct amount to avoid "unintentionally starving nonprofit organizations." Standish shared that her foundation has not formally changed its indirect policy, but it is interested in analyses of the true costs for their partners and in understanding how to support them in strengthening the sustainability of the work.

Reflecting on earlier mentions of "power building," Meadows commented that the phrase can unintentionally connote that the foundation is giving something—power—to the grantee, and that narrative can be problematic. An audience question, Meadows added, stated that although philanthropy, unlike government, responded to the crisis, the private-sector response is not sustainable, so what should the role of government be, and is "power building in individual communities fast enough or forward enough to make the changes?" Martinez Garcel remarked that the right framing is "unleash the power" because "we know the power is there," and what philanthropy can do is create "the opportunity for people to move together and move powerfully together." But that in itself is not enough unless policies, systems, and organizations show they value community input and integrate community suggestions in policy and systems, and organizations become aligned to respond to the effects of "centuries of disinvestment of communities of color." She added that investments in the sense of agency are needed, and she hopes that is surfacing in order to influence changes in government policy. Martinez Garcel added:

> People need to own and seek out solutions they want to see happening. I want to see young people that are organizing movements in city council positions and run for Senate positions. I want to see them be the ones who write the laws and sit in places where judges sit right now to define a case of a police officer versus a Black woman who is murdered in her home. That's what we need to do. I'm not looking at this to happen tomorrow but in this generation. We have to accelerate. Yes, it is enough. Yes, it is what we have to do now to have the sustainable changes we all want to see.

With regard to changing the sector, Martinez Garcel asserted that philanthropic organizations need to write their commitments into bylaws and policies, including reflecting the racial diversity of the communities they are serving. For example, her organization devotes 20 percent of grant making "to unleash the power of communities of color."

Standish said that two actions are needed in order to unleash the power of communities. First, the field needs to become faster at grant making and spending more, including connecting grantees to a larger ecosystem, such as with data-generating efforts and legal assistance. Secondly, the field needs to strengthen the work of "unleashing the power with long-term leadership commitment, building the pipeline, [and] building the places and opportunities where organizers, advocates, and policy makers can connect and strategize and plan."

Green commented that it is important to think of this work of unleashing power not as a project grant, a program, an organization, or even for an individual leader, but rather, as a long-term, sustained, and well-supported movement. Referring to advocacy work, Green underscored the need to fund community advocacy in the way that philanthropy has funded large traditional advocacy organizations.

Larkin added the element of evidence and evaluation to the conversation, but noted that evaluation needs to be equitable and designed together with grantees. A paradigm shift is needed to inform how philanthropy supports grantees in conducting good data collection, analysis, and evaluation to help unleash community power and support civic engagement and positive changes in communities.

Meadows shared another question from the audience pertaining to how values inform an organization's investments. Martinez Garcel spoke to programmatic investments in the community. More than 51 percent of her foundation's board and staff is Latino, and the organization invests 65 percent of the funds it pays out to organizations that have budgets that are below $1 million; that are grassroots, without the luxury of grant writers; and that are led by trusted community leaders with lived experience. In other words, this is about making sure that the money follows the institution's values. Larkin discussed the investment of a foundation's endowment, acknowledging that the sector has a history of investing in ways that have been detrimental to communities of color. The foundation is investing in affordable housing and other work that advances health equity and racial equity, and those considerations are applied across all of the foundation's work.

Green noted that her foundation uses some program-related investing, which offers low-interest loans to community-based organizations as well as larger institutions, to allow the foundation to grow its resources for greater effect. The foundation also applies the lens of environmental, social, and governance (ESG) questions to its investments to ensure alignment with its values. Moreover, it is working to ensure that more of the people who manage its investments are women and people of color. Because her foundation has the vast majority of its resources in an endowment and not in grants, it holds "the money, power, and decision making" and is exploring ways to enable communities to have agency over resources. Standish added that her foundation also uses the strategies described by others, from ESG to diversity among investment managers, as well as program-related investments—all of which can help move the field of investment capital toward being a more equitable field.

Meadows shared another question from the audience. Are foundations extractive capitalists, and what are workshop participants' organizations doing to ensure that they are accountable to the community? Buster responded that it is essential that foundations bring all of their resources and assets to bear in their support of communities. As an example, if a foundation is supporting a rural, low-income community, and foundation leaders have connections at the U.S. Department of Agriculture or with rural economic development practitioners, then "you have to bring those resources into the community—not just to grantees, but all the relationships you have." Martinez Garcel noted that the idea of philanthropy being extractive may be linked with the fact that although foundations are tax exempt, they may "sit" on large endowments. The fact that they only invest 5 percent of those resources is unjust when there are many ways that those resources could be invested. Being honest about philanthropy also requires acknowledging that the sector extracts ideas, knowledge, and human capital, and foundations may take too much credit for the work that communities are doing and the fact that communities are thriving. Also, when foundations invest in large firms to develop communication strategy and the narratives about the work, it must be acknowledged that the ideas they are putting forward are extracted from communities. While the communication firm is paid to come up with a solution or a logic model, the insights used are sourced from interviews with community organizers.

Standish shared The California Endowment's President's Youth Council as one strategy that the foundation uses to listen to the community. This group of young people also has a formal relationship with the board, which facilitates mutual understanding and better listening "to the voices of people who are most proximate to the experiences we are trying to address." Buster added that he observed that the Youth Council truly challenges the foundation's leadership, and he shared his view that more leaders would benefit from being open to working with the community in that way.

Larkin built on the earlier theme of philanthropy working with and creating with communities versus being extractive. "Philanthropy has a long history of reaching in the community and not giving back or not showing up in a way that elevates the solutions that are coming from community," she said. Listening and understanding communities and working to create "learning networks that people can tap into" is important.

The last question from the audience that Meadows shared asked if any foundations are exploring ways to support grantees similar to an endowment so that they do not have to apply for funding each year. Buster responded that he has been fighting for that for 15 years, but has not seen it happen. However, he noted, this is an issue for the philanthropic sector to consider, even if he has not seen much movement on it. Larkin agreed and said that she has not seen that type of support constitute a long-term solution.

Standish said that her organization has rarely used this approach, and in her experience, it did not work very well. She also made two additional points. Some of the foundation's working program-related investments (PRIs) are not exactly endowments, but they are intended to be mechanisms to help nonprofit organizations develop assets such as owning their own buildings. Thus, PRIs can be an important resource that grantees can use over time. The California Endowment makes mostly 2-year grants, Standish noted, and she asked if others make longer grants. How can foundations shift their thinking toward the longer term to facilitate sustainability, despite the many challenges of longer grants? Larkin stated that one of the strategies in use is general operating support, which may include longer duration grants, but impact investing, supervised guarantees, or low-market loans are other ways that the philanthropy sector can be more supportive in terms of long-term health and sustainability.

Meadows offered panelists a final chance to share. Martinez Garcel described how her foundation, which focuses on the largest ethnic population in California, is working to increase its endowment while also sharing with communities, and shifting generational wealth. The foundation views its work as investing in organizations led by people of color with a long-term focus, building the asset base to allow grantees to have more security to do the work they are doing for generations to come, and to stay in their locations without having to worry about rent increases for their facilities. Growing the endowment is critically important for organizations led by people of color who will build the pipeline of future civic and political leaders. Buster's closing comment was "know who you are centering in your work, know who you network with, and use [that knowledge] to the extent you can."

7

Insights and Strategies from Cross-Sector Thinkers

The objective of the cross-sector panel was to highlight the perspectives of individuals working at the intersection of different sectors and who are knowledgeable about data, actions, and policies, including investments outside of the health sector or at the interface among sectors, that have implications for improving equitable health and well-being in communities around the country. Mary Pittman, president and chief executive officer of the Public Health Institute, welcomed and introduced the panel: Chris Parker from the Georgia Health Policy Center (GHPC); Alison Omens from JUST Capital; and Soma Saha from Well-being and Equity in the World (WE in the World). Key points from the panelists are provided in Box 7-1.

Pittman asked the panelists to talk about the work of their organizations and how the pandemic and movement for racial justice are reshaping their work. Chris Parker shared two concepts. First, he said he would reflect on the work of GHPC on wellness funds, how stakeholder groups across the country are thinking about financing to support community health improvement, and the effects of the pandemic on that work, whether as a catalyst or as a factor in some unraveling of the partnership. A second area is alignment across sectors, particularly public health, health care, and the social sector, and how COVID-19 has affected that alignment. Parker also clarified that when he says COVID-19, he is using it as shorthand for the triple threat of pandemic, economic downturn, and the light that the pandemic has shed on racial inequality and inequities in the United States. The threat posed by racial inequities has been known for some time, Parker

45

BOX 7-1
Key Points from Individual Panelists

- Putting in practice an organizational commitment to being antiracist requires both internally and externally facing work. For the latter, those considerations need to inform contracting, hiring, procurement, and other aspects of the organization. (Parker)
- For companies, the CEO Blueprint for Racial Equity recommends (1) transparency about internal aspects from hiring to advancement to training; (2) considering community impact, including in philanthropy and in relationships with government and others; and (3) assessing societal effects of lobbying, advocacy, and the nature of corporate investments. (Omens)
- Community capacity building, trust, and a focus on equity have been a common ingredient in collaborative efforts that have been able to respond to the current crisis with resilience and effectiveness. However, trust takes time, and shortcuts for the sake of speed are unhelpful. (Saha)

---

noted, but the pandemic has cast it into sharp relief and that may help move the conversation forward.

Pittman asked Parker to speak about wellness funds. Most people, Parker began, understand that the U.S. health care delivery system is designed so that a lot is paid for sickness care. Communities have to gather resources in an effort to try to move upstream, or in other words, to address the underlying factors that shape health. Five to 10 years ago, GHPC became aware of innovations happening across the country as people were thinking about how to sustainably finance the work of community health improvement. Local wellness funds are "funds that are put together in an effort to address a local community priority" pertaining to health and well-being. GHPC has been working to understand how these funds work and the extent to which they are either site-specific or have features that could be scaled and replicated elsewhere.

Omens shared how her organization, a nonprofit founded approximately 7 years ago, works "to understand how Americans feel about companies and align corporate actions with those priorities." JUST Capital, she stated, conducts "extensive polling of what Americans think is important for companies to be prioritizing every day." The current top issues are worker pay, benefits, training, and commitment to nondiscrimination and advancement. Additional priorities include impact on climate and the environment, and consumer privacy, but a considerable proportion of the priorities have to do with health outcomes. JUST Capital reviews a variety of publicly available and crowdsourced data and information about the 1,000 largest publicly traded companies on those priority elements.

In the past 2 to 3 years, Omens said, there has been a move in the direction of stakeholder capitalism,[1] a concept that reflects a company's commitment not simply to shareholders, but to workers, communities, and consumers, as well as a company's impact on the environment. In a larger context where trust in institutions has broken down, Omens asserted, it is interesting to note a level of public faith in businesses as societal leaders. For example, she shared that consumers are asking for things that are not simply for profit but also offer long-term returns.

During the pandemic, consumers are asking if companies have implemented hazard pay and if they have kept it, and if they have sick leave and what the parameters are for it with regard to COVID-19 (e.g., is testing required; paid versus unpaid). JUST Capital, Omens noted, reflects on the profiles of companies that represent more than 20 million Americans, and has been asking companies a wide range of questions. One line of questioning may begin with if the company has assessed its workforce to ask if workers are able to get by economically, and explored why or why not. It is understood that if someone is financially insecure—because their wages are too low, their health care, transportation, or housing costs are too high, or their children are experiencing an illness—then it affects the business and productivity may be affected. Similarly, "If people don't feel respected on the job, they don't feel like they have a voice on the job," this has implications for the community, families, and the broader workforce.

Omens shared that JUST Capital frames the narrative about leadership as "doing well by workers" (with attention to better societal outcomes) as opposed to having the most buybacks or dividends. Pittman asked about key current findings among the companies tracked. Omens shared the example of Home Depot, which JUST Capital found gave workers adequate sick leave. Some companies that employ so-called essential workers offered hazard pay at the beginning of the pandemic, but many have discontinued it. The ramifications of the pandemic, however, are noteworthy if stores are located in places where there are outbreaks or if there are problems with the supply chain.

Pittman then asked Soma Saha to share the work of WE in the World and the Well Being In the Nation (WIN) Network. Two years ago, Saha said, nearly 100 organizations came together to work on the measures that were designed as a living library of measures, as reflected in the recent *Milbank Quarterly* article that showed how the measures were being used in the field (Saha et al., 2020). The *Milbank Quarterly* article describes frameworks and tools being used to advance equity, racial justice, and well-being measurement in real time in states ranging from Delaware to

---

[1] See https://hbr.org/2020/01/making-stakeholder-capitalism-a-reality (accessed January 13, 2021).

Texas.[2] A major lesson is that the systems are not working, and "we need one another." A key insight shared by participants is that they need help both in thinking about how to effect inner transformation while also working toward structural transformation. Saha also mentioned contributing to *Thriving Together: Springboard for Equitable Recovery and Resilience*,[3] a guide and list of web resources from the Well-Being Trust and supported by the Centers for Disease Control and Prevention Foundation, and highlighting key actions that communities can take to move through recovering from COVID-19 and toward health, well-being, and equity.

Pittman asked the panelists to share what they have learned about advancing equitable health and well-being over the years through cross-sector work. Pittman remarked on the effects of COVID-19 on Black and Latino communities and asked the panelists to speak about what they are observing in terms of cross-sector work in advancing equitable health and racial equity as part of the response to the pandemic. Omens shared that JUST Capital partnered with PolicyLink and the consulting firm FSG to develop the CEO Blueprint for Racial Equity, and outlined its three main recommendations.[4] First, the blueprint calls on companies to be transparent about what they are doing internally, including the demographics, assessment on hiring and opportunities for advancement, and leadership training on antiracism. Second, the blueprint recommends that companies think about their effects in their community, including changing their approach to philanthropy and their relationships with local governments, organizations, and suppliers. Third, the blueprint asks companies to consider their effects at a societal level and in terms of lobbying and advocacy. For example, Omens said, "If you are a bank or you have capital, where is that capital flowing? Have you done an assessment of it?" There are considerably limitations to currently available public data on these topics, Omens noted, because companies generally do not share demographic data or data on their board diversity, but, she added, there is a real push both within companies at the board level and through investors asking for those data. Given the current context, Omens said that it will be important for the corporate sector to find ways to measure "what it means to be a company committed to antiracism."

Parker shared that the antiracism question is a personal issue for him. He shared his sense of indescribable rage after seeing the Ahmaud Arbery

---

[2] See https://www.milbank.org/quarterly/articles/well-being-in-the-nation-a-living-library-of-measures-to-drive-multi-sector-population-health-improvement-and-address-social-determinants (accessed December 18, 2022).

[3] See https://wellbeingtrust.org/news/well-being-trust-releases-thriving-together-a-springboard-for-equitable-recovery-and-resilience-in-communities-across-america (accessed December 18, 2022).

[4] See https://www.policylink.org/resources-tools/ceo-blueprint-for-racial-equity (accessed December 18, 2022).

videotape, and coming to acknowledge that the question about antiracism is both organizational and personal. The components of this work include "do no harm" at the organizational level, the personal emotional intelligence to recognize that this is not merely a technical challenge, and also the need to consider and adopt multiple strategies. Change, Parker noted, needs to occur at all levels: internally in the organization, at the level of the partnerships in which the organization participates, and externally facing at the societal level to avoid perpetuating something that has been structural or systemic. Questions to be asked, according to Parker, should touch on contracting, hiring, and other aspects of the organization. Organizations outside health care, such as public health and the social sector, may believe that power resides in the health care system, and it is important to address that power dynamic. GHPC, Parker added, has begun thinking about the tools needed to help organizations sustain these conversations about race and power.

The WE in the Nation meeting after the killing of George Floyd, Saha stated, surfaced what seemed to be a moral crisis in people's minds regarding how to act. WE in the Nation invited people to a dialogue facilitated by members of communities of color and groups with relevant experience to help co-create what became the WE WIN Together Racial Justice Journey. Saha echoed Parker's remarks that relationships need to change and power dynamics need to be addressed as organizations set out "to transform our policies, our investments, our practices, our system, our culture."

Pittman asked the speakers to describe one or two strategies for responding to the pandemic and the movement for justice that they have found to be effective. Saha shared that her organization has been working to gather links for resources and has disseminated them on the WE in the World website, on Community Commons, and elsewhere. Saha also shared an insight from the racial justice community—that accompaniment matters and that people who feel energized and motivated after a training or conference will need day-to-day support and a group of peers to walk with them on their journey. Saha also shared that Transformation 2020 from the Center for Popular Democracy was starting the following day.

Parker added that partnerships across organizations require additional support that is different from what is needed for internal, institutional work and for outward-facing work.

Funders and organizations such as GHPC provide support to some of these cross-sector collaborations. For example, Parker mentioned that the Atlanta City Council approached GHPC for help with facilitating the council's own conversations about racial equity and bringing information and tools to the council table.

Omens spoke from the perspective of business, and echoed the questions about cross-sector partnerships. JUST Capital works to understand, for example, what a company's policy is on its relationship with the community, how it chooses where to spend its philanthropic dollars, or how it chooses to hire. Omens added that JUST Capital has been experimenting with content and creating lists, such as "10 things businesses can do right now to support essential workers or to promote racial equity," which has gotten considerable attention on Google and other search engines.

Pittman asked Parker to respond to an audience question about supporting Accountable Communities for Health. Even though many have been successful in building strong, cross-sector collaboratives, had Parker observed in his research any strong, sustainable funding commitments that he could share? What would it take to make that kind of investment or that change in financing happen so these local collaboratives can be sustained over time?

Parker acknowledged that over the past 5 years, there has been greater interest and engagement of health systems in population health, perhaps from an initial standpoint of "How do I make the bottom line feel better?" or "How do I take care of our patients and not necessarily the broader community?" Some of this work has been led by the mission-oriented hospital systems, and some of the conversations about the power imbalance have come from health systems being at the table. Then, COVID-19 happened, and it is unclear what the effect has been aside from destabilizing the finances of health systems.

Parker noted that the opportunity presented by COVID-19 may be overshadowed by the need to stanch the bleeding, and a second wave of COVID-19 may further affect the appetite of health systems to engage in this work rather than work on improving hospital infrastructure. Parker also outlined the framework for what GHPC describes as alignment:

- trust and power,
- power distribution,
- data sharing,
- a common vision, and
- sitting together at the table for the good of the community.

The groups that are working toward sustainability, Parker noted, are the groups that are working through these issues. Saha shared an observation that partnerships that have co-invested in community capacity building and that have approached the work with equity in mind have been able to develop far greater resilience and preparedness in their ability to solve problems. However, she added, in aiming to do good quickly, some collaborators have made some other sectors serve the ends or align with the approaches of the health care system, she added. She said,

> That actually is not productive because it is way more costly and super inefficient, and it also overwhelms the health system itself. I think the same can be said for large businesses that [are] major employer[s].

Saha underscored the value of achieving some quick wins. For example, in work taking place in San Antonio, where 60 percent of children did not have an Internet connection for virtual learning, the effort to improve access for telemedicine became a broader effort for jobs and community health. However, Saha noted that "you can't shortcut that recipe if you're actually going to create well-being and equity out of that well-being trust. The trust is an enabler ... and the communities that approach it in that way achieve far better outcomes."

Pittman shared the unique opportunity that the Public Health Institute has as a result of 12 California foundations coming together to fund COVID-19 contact tracing work in high-impact communities. The funders organized the work rapidly in response to the pandemic, and, she added, there may be other examples of such unlikely but exemplary rapid responses to the pandemic.

Omens remarked that people are seeing a shift in the business community in real time. Adding to her earlier comment about stakeholder capitalism, Omens noted that the Business Roundtable signed a new statement of purpose in August 2019, saying that the purpose of business is not just to their shareholders but to their workers and communities and suppliers. There are questions, Omens said, such as "Does business have a role to play in addressing inequality? If the retail and restaurant industry are paying really low wages, is that a business question? Is that a question for business operations?" The sector may begin to see collaborations that are just about philanthropic dollars going to local sports teams shift to conversations about "aligning investments along with philanthropy, along with paying living wages, and you can start to see the outcomes that are connected in a whole different set of ways," Omens added.

Parker shared that a topic that he has encountered in his work that pertains to the role of public health vis-à-vis health care is the sense that "the public sector acquiesces the role of leadership to the private sector." The (governmental) public health role of connector between the health care system and the community at large is important, Parker noted. He acknowledged that the leadership role in a community health improvement partnership could be played by any number of entities, from a health care organization to a social services agency. However, he noted that public health workers and officials have traditionally acted as facilitators of leadership and data gatherers or data sharers in the community, and although (governmental) public health as the go-to-source for credible information has been imperiled somewhat, there is a unique role that public health plays that may not be easily be transferred to other entities.[5]

_____

[5] See the description of public health agencies as the community's "chief health strategist" that has shaped the field's thinking about the current and potential role of government public health agencies at https://www.resolve.ngo/docs/the-high-achieving-governmental-

Pittman said that she would agree, and then asked Saha to reflect. Saha said that she "would love to see public health, which brings that ability to see across sectors, be the coordinating entity." She appreciated what Pittman had shared about community health workers in the context of COVID-19 operating not just as COVID-19 tracers, but rather

> as people who both know and have relationships with the community, understanding people's well-being overall and the community's well-being, and contributors to the planning process for what actually needs to shift and grow, and invest[ing] in them as community leaders would be something I would love to see happen as we emerge out of this pandemic so that we really have that power.

Saha noted that the public sector is uniquely positioned to create an enabling policy environment. For example, she described how a policy environment could provide incentives, such as tax benefits, for "businesses that measured their contribution to the well-being of their people, the well-being of community, and their investments [in] racial justice."

health-department-as-the-chief-health-strategist-by-2020-final1636869407709140046.pdf (accessed January 13, 2021).

Appendix A

References

Costello, E. J., W. Copeland, and A. Angold. 2016. The Great Smoky Mountains Study: Developmental epidemiology in the southeastern United States. *Social Psychiatry and Psychiatric Epidemiology* 51(5):639–646.

EPIP (Emerging Practitioners in Philanthropy). 2018. *Dissonance & disconnects: How entry and mid-level foundation staff see their futures, their institutions, and their field*. http://racial equity.issuelab.org/resources/33121/33121.pdf (accessed December 18, 2022).

Gollust, S. E., J. Niederdeppe, and C. L. Barry. 2013. Framing the consequences of childhood obesity to increase public support for obesity prevention policy. *American Journal of Public Health* 103(11):e96–e102.

Hardeman, H., and J. Karbeah. 2020. Examining racism in health services research: A disciplinary self critique. *Health Services Research* 55(S2):777–780.

Kindig, D., and G. Stoddart. 2003. What is population health? *American Journal of Public Health* 93(3):380–383.

IOM (Institute of Medicine). 2003. *Unequal treatment: Confronting racial and ethnic disparities in health care*. Washington, DC: The National Academies Press.

NASEM (National Academies of Sciences, Engineering, and Medicine). 2017. *Accounting for social risk factors in Medicare payment*. Washington, DC: The National Academies Press https://nap.nationalacademies.org/resource/23605/interactive (accessed January 9, 2023).

NASEM. 2018. *Learning through citizen science: Enhancing opportunities by design*. Washington, DC: The National Academies Press.

Rifkin, S. B. 2003. A framework linking community empowerment and health equity: It is a matter of CHOICE. *Journal of Health, Population, and Nutrition* 21(3):168–180.

Saha, S., B. B. Cohen, J. Nagy, M. E. McPherson, and R. Phillips. 2020. *Well-being in the nation: A living library of measures to drive multi-sector population health improvement and address social determinants*. https://onlinelibrary.wiley.com/doi/full/10.1111/1468-0009.12477 (accessed February 11, 2021).

Trust for America's Health. 2020. *The impact of chronic underfunding on America's public health system: Trends, risks, and recommendations, 2020.* https://www.tfah.org/report-details/publichealthfunding2020 (accessed December 18, 2022).

Tsai, J., L. Ucik, N. Baldwin, C. Hasslinger, and P. George. 2016. MHPE race matters? Examining and rethinking race portrayal in preclinical medical education. *Academic Medicine* 91(7):916–920.

Appendix B

Workshop Agenda

Monday, September 21

11:00 a.m.–
12:30 p.m. EDT

Academic Public Health and Population Health Session

Sandro Galea, Boston University
Marc Gourevitch, New York University Langone Health
Dora Hughes, The George Washington University
Sheri Johnson, University of Wisconsin–Madison
Shreya Kangovi, University of Pennsylvania
Ziad Obermeyer, University of California, Berkeley
Joshua Sharfstein, Johns Hopkins University (*moderator*)

1:30 p.m.–
3:00 p.m. EDT

Social Sector Session

Cathy Baase, Michigan Health Improvement Alliance
Susan Dreyfus, Alliance for Strong Families and Communities
Gary Gunderson, Wake Forest Baptist Health and Wake Forest University

Milton Little, United Way of Greater Atlanta
 (*moderator*)
Jason Purnell, BJC Healthcare and Washington
 University in St. Louis

Tuesday, September 22

11:00 a.m.–
12:30 p.m. EDT

Health Care Session

Philip Alberti, Association of American Medical
 Colleges
Dawn Alley, U.S. Department of Health and Human
 Services
Kirsten Bibbins-Domingo, University of California,
 San Francisco
Sanne Magnan, HealthPartners Institute
 (*moderator*)
Von Nguyen, Blue Cross Blue Shield of North
 Carolina
Stella Whitney-West, NorthPoint Health and
 Wellness

3:30 p.m.–
5:00 p.m. EDT

Public Health Session

John Auerbach, Trust for America's Health
 (*moderator*)
Oxiris Barbot, formerly New York City Department
 of Health and Mental Hygiene
Joneigh Khaldun, Michigan Department of Health
 and Human Services
José Montero, Centers for Disease Control and
 Prevention
Umair Shah, Harris County Public Health
Monica Valdes Lupi, The Kresge Foundation

Wednesday, September 23

1:30 p.m.–
3:00 p.m. EDT

Cross-Sector Session

Alison Omens, JUST Capital
Chris Parker, Georgia Health Policy Center
Mary Pittman, Public Health Institute (moderator)
Soma Saha, Well Being In the Nation Network

Thursday, September 24

11:00 a.m.–
12:30 p.m. EDT

Philanthropy Session

William Buster, St. David's Foundation
Rose Green, Colorado Health Foundation
Michelle Larkin, Robert Wood Johnson Foundation
Jacqueline Martinez Garcel, Latino Community
    Foundation
Phyllis Meadows, The Kresge Foundation
    (*moderator*)
Marion Standish, The California Endowment

Appendix C

Speaker and Planning Committee Member Biosketches

Dawn Alley, Ph.D., is the chief strategy officer at the Center for Medicare & Medicaid Innovation (CMMI). She previously served as the deputy senior advisor for Value-based Transformation in the Office of the Secretary of the U.S. Department of Health and Human Services, and as the director of the Prevention and Population Health Group at CMMI, which is responsible for innovative payment and service delivery models including the Accountable Health Communities model, the Million Hearts Cardiovascular Risk Reduction model, and the Medicare Diabetes Prevention Program. Prior to joining CMMI, Dr. Alley served as the senior advisor in the Office of the Surgeon General, where she oversaw implementation of the National Prevention Strategy. She has extensive expertise in population health and aging, with more than 50 publications in journals including the *New England Journal of Medicine* and *JAMA*. Dr. Alley holds a Ph.D. in gerontology from the University of Southern California and received postdoctoral training in population health through the Robert Wood Johnson Foundation Health and Society Scholars program at the University of Pennsylvania.

Philip Alberti, Ph.D., is the senior director for health equity research and policy at the Association of American Medical Colleges (AAMC). He supports the efforts of academic medical centers to build an evidence base for effective programs, protocols, and partnerships aimed at ameliorating inequalities in health and health care through research. Dr. Alberti is responsible for working with AAMC's constituents to elevate the status of community-partnered and health equity–related research efforts, iden-

tifying emerging funding sources and policy implications for such projects, and disseminating findings to achieve the broadest possible impact.
Prior to joining AAMC in 2012, Dr. Alberti led research, evaluation, and
planning efforts for a bureau within the New York City Department of
Health and Mental Hygiene that works to promote health equity between
disadvantaged and advantaged neighborhoods. Dr. Alberti holds a Ph.D.
in sociomedical sciences from the Columbia University Mailman School
of Public Health and was a National Institute of Mental Health Fellow in
the Psychiatric Epidemiology Training program.

John Auerbach, M.B.A., is the president and the chief executive officer
of Trust for America's Health (TFAH), a nonprofit, nonpartisan organization dedicated to saving lives by protecting the health of every community and working to make disease prevention a national priority. TFAH
conducts science-based research, issues policy-oriented reports addressing key health issues, shares best practices from communities large and
small across the nation, and brings diverse groups together to effectively
respond to current and emerging health threats of all kinds.

Mr. Auerbach was formerly the associate director for policy and the
acting director of the Office for State, Tribal, Local, and Territorial Support at the Centers for Disease Control and Prevention (CDC). As such,
he managed CDC's Policy Office, which focused on strengthening the
collaboration between the public health and health care sectors, and he
oversaw key activities and technical assistance that supported the nation's
health departments and the public health system. Prior to his appointment at CDC, he was a Distinguished Professor of Practice in Health
Sciences and the director of the Institute on Urban Health Research and
Practice at Northeastern University from 2012 to 2014.

He was the commissioner of public health for the Commonwealth of
Massachusetts from 2007 to 2012. He participated in the implementation
of the state's innovative health care reform law and developed public
health programs that promoted health equity, emergency preparedness,
and chronic and infectious disease prevention. Prior to his appointment as
commissioner, Mr. Auerbach had been the executive director of the Boston
Public Health Commission for 9 years. In this position he oversaw a wide
range of city services including those addressing substance abuse, home-
lessness, and emergency medical services. He had previously worked at
the State Health Department for a decade, first as the chief of staff and
later as an assistant commissioner overseeing the HIV/AIDS Bureau during the early years of the epidemic.

Cathy Baase, M.D., serves as the board chair of the Michigan Health
Improvement Alliance (MIHIA), a multistakeholder collaborative dedi-

cated to improving the health of people in 14 counties of central Michigan. In a related role, she is the senior fellow serving MIHIA and the transformational Transforming Health Regionally in a Vibrant Economy initiative. She is a member of the Roundtable on Population Health Improvement of the National Academies of Sciences, Engineering, and Medicine, and she served as the initial chair of the Business Collaborative. Dr. Baase is a member of the Stewardship Council of Raising the Bar, an initiative funded by the Robert Wood Johnson Foundation (RWJF) to set bold new principles for the role that health care systems and institutions should play in achieving optimal health and well-being, and practical guidance for applying them. Additionally, she is a member of the National Alliance to Impact Social Determinants of Health and serves as a senior advisor to HealthBegins, which is focused on upstream efforts in health care. Dr. Baase is a member of the Advisory Council for the RWJF Culture of Health for Business project with the Global Reporting Index. She is also on the Susan and Henry Samueli College of Health Sciences Advisory Board at the University of California, Irvine.

Oxiris Barbot, M.D., has more than 25 years of experience in public health and health care delivery and has dedicated her career to achieving health equity. When she was the commissioner of health for New York City, she led the nation's premier health department in centering an equity agenda on communities, bridging public health and health care delivery, and leveraging data for action and policy. She successfully navigated the city's responses to the first wave of the COVID-19 pandemic and to New York City's largest measles outbreak in 30 years.

As an innovative public health leader, Dr. Barbot has championed addressing health inequities in major cities along the East Coast. In 2010, Dr. Barbot was appointed the commissioner of health for the City of Baltimore. During her tenure in Baltimore, she led the development of Healthy Baltimore 2015, a robust health agenda dedicated to ensuring that all Baltimore residents realize their full health potential. Under her leadership, the City of Baltimore achieved a record reduction in the rate of infant deaths, among many achievements in health. From 2003 to 2010, Dr. Barbot served as the medical director of New York City's public schools. In this capacity, she spearheaded development and implementation of an electronic health record system that improved delivery of health services for more than 1 million children. Prior to her work in New York City, Dr. Barbot served as the chief of pediatrics and community medicine at Unity Health Care, Inc., a federally qualified health center in Washington, DC. Dr. Barbot holds a bachelor's degree from Yale University and an M.D. from the University of Medicine and Dentistry of New Jersey. She completed her pediatric residency at The George Washington University's Children's National Medical Center.

Kirsten Bibbins-Domingo, Ph.D., M.D., M.A.S., is a professor and the chair of the Department of Epidemiology and Biostatistics and the Lee Goldman, M.D., Endowed Chair and Professor of Medicine at the University of California, San Francisco (USCF). She is the inaugural vice dean for population health and health equity in the UCSF School of Medicine. She co-founded the UCSF Center for Vulnerable Populations at Zuckerberg San Francisco General Hospital that focuses on actionable research to increase health equity and reduce health disparities in at-risk communities. She is one of the Principal Investigators for the UCSF Clinical and Translational Sciences Institute, and she leads the newly launched UCSF COVID Community Public Health Initiative.

Dr. Bibbins-Domingo is a general internist and cardiovascular epidemiologist whose scholarship includes observational epidemiology, pragmatic trials, and simulation modeling to examine clinical and public health approaches to prevention in the United States and globally. She previously served on and led the United States Preventive Services Task Force from 2010 to 2017. She is an inducted member of the American Society for Clinical Investigation, the Association of American Physicians, and the National Academy of Medicine.

William Buster, M.A., is the executive vice president of community investments at the St. David's Foundation. He leads and oversees the Foundation's grantmaking and community programs, including the St. David's Dental Program. Prior to joining the Foundation in 2016, Mr. Buster was the owner and lead consultant for Common-Unity Philanthropic and Nonprofit Advisors. He also worked with the W.K. Kellogg Foundation, where he served as the director of Mississippi and New Orleans Programs as well as an advisor to the president on Men and Boys of Color, and as a program officer with the Mary Reynolds Babcock Foundation, with a focus on Arkansas, Louisiana, Mississippi, Tennessee, and parts of Appalachia. Earlier in his career, he was the program director for community development for the Greensboro Education and Development Council. Mr. Buster has an M.A. in policy and practice of development from the University of New Hampshire, and a B.A. from North Carolina Agricultural & Technical University.

Nupur Chaudhury, M.P.H., M.U.P., is the program officer of the New York State Health Foundation (NYSHealth). She focuses on NYSHealth's priority area on building healthy communities, which leads neighborhood-level and policy interventions to increase residents' access to healthy, affordable food options; improve the built environment; and link communities with healthy lifestyle programming. Ms. Chaudhury has a background in community-based health, urban planning, and community organizing.

Prior to joining NYSHealth, Ms. Chaudhury was the director of neighborhood health development at the Center for Health Equity, New York City Department of Health and Mental Hygiene. In her role there, she led the expansion of the Shop Healthy program, aimed at changing the food retail environment in the city's poorest neighborhoods, and she was also part of the planning team developing the city's Neighborhood Health Action Centers. She has also worked with Rebuild by Design as a resiliency planner after Hurricane Sandy by building and strengthening neighborhood coalitions in Connecticut, New Jersey, and New York. Prior to that, Ms. Chaudhury was the first health coordinator for the Brownsville Partnership, developing its agenda linking the built environment, health, and violence to its work on active living and healthy eating. Ms. Chaudhury holds a B.A. from Bryn Mawr College, an M.U.P. from New York University, and an M.P.H. from Columbia University. She is a member of the American Public Health Association and the American Planning Association and also serves on the boards of Made in Brownsville and University of Orange.

Susan N. Dreyfus is the president and the chief executive officer (CEO) of the Alliance for Strong Families and Communities, a strategic action network of social-sector organizations that has a national reach in thousands of communities across America. Prior to joining the Alliance in 2012, Ms. Dreyfus was the secretary for the Washington State Department of Social and Health Services. She was appointed by Governor Chris Gregoire in May 2009 and approved by the senate, and she served as a member of the Governor's Executive Cabinet. She had responsibility for Medicaid, aging and long-term care, child welfare, behavioral health care, juvenile justice, economic assistance, and other human services. Before her work in Washington state, Ms. Dreyfus served as the senior vice president and the chief operating officer for the Alliance.

In 1996 she was appointed by the Governor Tommy G. Thompson administration in Wisconsin to be the first administrator of the Division of Children and Family Services. Her responsibilities included child welfare, child care quality and licensing, youth development, and an array of emergency assistance and other community programs. Ms. Dreyfus is a member of Leadership 18, a coalition of CEOs from the largest and most respected nonprofit organizations in America, and was previously the chair. She serves on the governing boards of the American Public Human Services Association and Generations United. Ms. Dreyfus is also on the advisory committees of the Social Intervention Research & Evaluation Network and the Robert Wood Johnson Foundation Systems for Action. She was appointed through the speaker's office in the U.S. House of Representatives to serve on the National Commission to Eliminate Child Abuse and Neglect Fatalities from 2013 to 2015.

Sandro Galea, M.D., M.P.H., Dr.P.H., is a physician, epidemiologist, author, and the dean and the Robert A. Knox Professor at the Boston University School of Public Health. He previously held academic and leadership positions at Columbia University, the University of Michigan, and The New York Academy of Medicine. He has published extensively in the peer-reviewed literature, and is a regular contributor to a range of public media about the social causes of health, mental health, and the consequences of trauma. He has been listed as one of the most widely cited scholars in the social sciences. He is the chair of the board of the Association of Schools and Programs of Public Health and the past president of the Society for Epidemiologic Research and of the Interdisciplinary Association for Population Health Science. He is an elected member of the National Academy of Medicine. Dr. Galea has received several lifetime achievement awards. Dr. Galea holds an M.D. from the University of Toronto, graduate degrees from Harvard University and Columbia University, and an honorary doctorate from the University of Glasgow.

Marc N. Gourevitch, M.D., M.P.H., is the Muriel G. and George W. Singer Professor and the founding chair of the Department of Population Health at the New York University (NYU) Langone Medical Center. The focus of Dr. Gourevitch's work is on developing approaches that leverage both health care delivery and policy- and community-level interventions to advance the health of populations. Dr. Gourevitch leads the City Health Dashboard initiative, funded by the Robert Wood Johnson Foundation, to equip city and community leaders with an accurate understanding of the health of their populations, including its social, economic, and environmental drivers, to support population health improvement. He directs NYU Langone's participation in the New York City Clinical Data Research Network funded by the Patient-Centered Outcomes Research Institute. In other research, he focuses on improving health outcomes among drug users and other underserved populations, including by integrating pharmacological treatments for opioid and alcohol dependence into primary care. Dr. Gourevitch previously served as the founding director of NYU Langone Health's Division of General Internal Medicine, and led NYU Langone Health's Centers for Disease Control and Prevention–funded Fellowship in Medicine and Public Health Research. A graduate of Harvard College and Harvard Medical School, he trained in primary care/internal medicine at NYU and Bellevue Hospital and received his M.P.H. from the Columbia University Mailman School of Public Health.

Rose Green, M.N.P., is a program officer at the Colorado Health Foundation who works to bring health in reach for communities across northeastern Colorado. She is currently focused locally on Morgan County and the

East Colfax Corridor. Ms. Green is fueled by a lifelong passion for equity and nonprofit work, grounded in a desire to make nonprofits more effective and impactful. She is also the co-chair of Emerging Practitioners in Philanthropy—Colorado. Before starting at the Colorado Health Foundation, Ms. Green was a training specialist with the Colorado Department of Health Care Policy and Financing. She attended Pomona College as an undergraduate in nonprofit organizational and economic development, and received an M.N.P. from Regis University.

Gary Gunderson, D.Min., D.Div., M.Div., is the vice president for faith and health, a professor of public health sciences, and a professor of religion and the health of the public (at the Divinity School), Wake Forest Baptist Health and Wake Forest University School of Divinity. His degrees, which hide as much as they illuminate, are an undergraduate degree from Wake Forest University in history, an M.Div. at Emory University (with an honors thesis on economics, faith, and the hungry) and a D.Min. from the Interdenominational Theology Centre in Atlanta (with a thesis on boundary leadership). However, his real qualifications are some 40 years of life in incredibly rich webs of relationships with people working seriously in the areas of hunger/poverty and community development, public health, and more recently health care, all of which are in the boundary zone between people moving out of their exclusive faith identities. Dr. Gunderson is interested in organizational and community change and how people influence complex human systems to morph in the direction of greater vitality, decency, and justice. He worked for about 8 years at the Carter Center, where many of these ideas were developed, and the Emory University Rollins School of Public Health, then 7 years as a senior executive at Methodist LeBonheur Healthcare (a $1.5 billion faith-based hospital system in Memphis, Tennessee, one of the poorest cities in the United States). His current work focuses on helping this large system align its full institutional and human assets with its professed goal of advancing the health of the region.

Dora Hughes, M.D., M.P.H., is the associate research professor of health policy & management at the Milken Institute School of Public Health at The George Washington University, where her work focuses on the intersection of clinical and community health, social determinants of health, health equity, health care quality, and workforce. Previously, Dr. Hughes was a senior policy advisor at Sidley Austin, where she advised on regulatory and legislative matters in the life science industry. Prior to that, she served for nearly 4 years in the Obama administration as the counselor for science & public health to Secretary Kathleen Sebelius at the U.S. Department of Health and Human Services. Her areas of responsibility included implementation of public health and U.S. Food and Drug Administration (FDA)-related provisions of the Patient Protection and Affordable Care Act, as well as signature legislation for tobacco, Alzheimer's disease, and FDA reform. She served in leadership roles for several White House initiatives, including the Childhood Obesity Task Force, the President's Food Safety Working Group, the Committee on STEM Education, and Let's Move. Dr. Hughes began her career in health policy as a senior program officer at The Commonwealth Fund, and subsequently as the deputy director for the HELP Committee under Senator Edward M. Kennedy. She then served as the health policy advisor to former Senator Barack Obama. Dr. Hughes received a B.S. from Washington University, an M.D. from Vanderbilt University, and an M.P.H. from Harvard University. She completed her internal medicine residency at Brigham & Women's Hospital.

Sheri Johnson, Ph.D., is the director of the Population Health Institute; an associate professor in the Department of Population Health Sciences; and an associate director of community partnerships for the Prevention Research Center at the University of Wisconsin–Madison, School of Medicine and Public Health. Dr. Johnson has dedicated her 25-year career to partnering with children, families, community organizations, and systems to advance health and well-being. Awed by the resilience of individuals and communities, she is motivated to remove unfair obstacles and conditions that create and perpetuate health inequities. Dr. Johnson completed her undergraduate studies at Brown University, earned an M.A. and Ph.D. in clinical psychology at Boston University, and served as a clinical fellow in psychology at Harvard Medical School. She was previously the director of behavioral health at Milwaukee Health Services, Inc., a federally qualified health center, and served as the administrator and state health officer for the Wisconsin Division of Public Health. Immediately prior to joining the Population Health Institute, she was the associate professor of pediatrics at the Medical College of Wisconsin Center for Advancement of Underserved Children, where she collaborated with diverse stakeholders to address a broad range of real-world problems.

Shreya Kangovi, M.D., M.S.H.P., is an internist, pediatrician, and health policy researcher. She is a leading national expert on the use of community health workers—trusted laypeople from local communities—to improve population health. Her research also sheds light on patient perspectives on health and health care utilization. Dr. Kangovi is the founding executive director of the Penn Center for Community Health Workers, a national center of excellence dedicated to advancing health in low-income populations through effective community health worker programs. The center is a hub for ongoing research and development of best practices for community health workers. Dr. Kangovi led the team that designed IMPaCT, a standardized, scalable community health worker program that has been proven in three randomized controlled trials to improve chronic disease control, primary care access, mental health, and quality of care while reducing hospital admissions.

Joneigh S. Khaldun, M.D., M.P.H., is the chief medical executive and the chief deputy director for health for the Michigan Department of Health and Human Services (MDHHS). In these roles, she provides medical guidance for the State of Michigan and oversees the Public Health, Medical Services, Aging and Adult Services, and Behavioral Health and Developmental Disabilities administrations. Prior to her roles at MDHHS, she was the director and the health officer for the Detroit Health Department, where she oversaw a robust community-driven community health assessment, established a comprehensive reproductive health network, and led Detroit's response to the hepatitis A outbreak. In 2018, Dr. Khaldun was selected for the 40 Under 40 Leaders in Minority Health Award by the National Minority Quality Forum; she is also a fellow of the American College of Emergency Physicians.

Previously, Dr. Khaldun was the Baltimore City Health Department's chief medical officer, where she oversaw seven clinics and a laboratory and led efforts to address the opioid epidemic. She has held several local and national leadership positions, including as the director of the Center for Injury Prevention and Control at The George Washington University, the founder and the director of the Fellowship in Health Policy in the University of Maryland Department of Emergency Medicine, and as a fellow in the Obama administration's Office of Health Reform.

Dr. Khaldun has served on several national and local boards and committees that include the Commission on Health in Montgomery County, Maryland; Big Brothers Big Sisters of Metropolitan Detroit; the Detroit Urban Research Collaborative; the governor-appointed Michigan Public Health Advisory Council; and the Centers for Disease Control and Prevention Health Disparities Advisory Committee. She obtained her undergraduate degree from the University of Michigan, M.D. from the University of Pennsylvania Perelman School of Medicine, and an M.P.H. in health policy from The George Washington University. She completed her residency in emergency medicine at Kings County Hospital Center in Brooklyn, New York, where she served as the chief resident. She practices emergency medicine part-time at Henry Ford Hospital in Detroit.

Milton J. Little, Jr., M.A., became the first African American president of United Way of Greater Atlanta, the second-largest in the national system, in July 2007. Altogether, Mr. Little has helped raise more than $500 million for local community needs and priorities. Before joining United Way, he served as the chief operating officer and the interim president and the chief executive officer of the National Urban League. He graduated magna cum laude from Morehouse College with a B.A. in sociology and earned an M.A. in urban sociology and social policy from Columbia University.

He is a member of many boards and advisory committees, including the Center for Assessment and Policy Development. He also served as the past chair of the Southern Education Foundation, and the past vice chair of the board of directors for Ways to Work. He is a member of the Atlanta Mayoral Board of Service, the Commerce Club Operating Board, 100 Black Men of Atlanta, Leadership Atlanta Class of 2010, and the Rotary Club of Atlanta. He also serves on the Junior League of Atlanta Community Advisory Board, the University of Georgia Advisory Board for the J.W. Fanning Institute for Leadership Development, the Atlanta Speech School Board of Advisors, the Woodruff Arts Center Board of Trustees, Central Atlanta Progress, the Georgia Chamber of Commerce, the Georgia Early Education Alliance for Ready Students, Georgia's Older Adults Cabinet, Georgia's Children's Cabinet, the Hope Atlanta Advisory Council, the Get Georgia Ready Reading Cabinet, and Susan G. Komen of Greater Atlanta. In January 2018, he was selected to serve on Mayor Keisha Lance Bottoms's Transition Team.

Sanne Magnan, M.D., Ph.D., is the co-chair of the Roundtable on Population Health Improvement of the National Academies of Sciences, Engineering, and Medicine. She is the former president and the chief executive officer of the Institute for Clinical Systems Improvement (2006–2007, 2011–2016). In 2007, she was appointed the commissioner of the Minnesota Department of Health by Minnesota Governor Tim Pawlenty. She served from 2007 to 2010 and had significant responsibility for the implementation of Minnesota's 2008 health reform legislation, including the Statewide Health Improvement Program, standardized quality reporting, development of provider peer grouping, certification process for health care homes, and baskets of care.

Dr. Magnan was a staff physician at the Tuberculosis Clinic at St. Paul–Ramsey County Department of Public Health (2002–2015). She was a member of the Population-based Payment Model Workgroup of the Healthcare Payment Learning and Action Network (2015–2016) and a member of the Centers for Medicare & Medicaid Services' Multisector Collaboration Measure Development Technical Expert Panel (2016). She is on Epic's Population Health Steering Board and on the Healthy People 2030 Engagement Subcommittee.

She served on the board of Minnesota Community Measurement and the board of NorthPoint Health & Wellness Center, a federally qualified health center and part of Hennepin Health. Her previous experience also includes serving as the vice president and the medical director of consumer health at the Blue Cross and Blue Shield of Minnesota. Currently, she is a senior fellow with HealthPartners Institute, and adjunct assistant professor of medicine at the University of Minnesota. Dr. Magnan holds an M.D. and a Ph.D. in medicinal chemistry from the University of Minnesota, and is a board-certified internist.

Jacqueline Martinez Garcel, M.P.H., is the chief executive officer of the Latino Community Foundation (LCF). The mission of LCF is to unleash the power of Latinos in California. She has led LCF through a critical stage of growth and expansion. Today, LCF leads one of the largest networks of Latino philanthropists in the country and it is the only statewide foundation solely focused on investing in Latino leaders. She is driven by a sense of urgency, justice, and determination to create opportunities for Latinos to thrive economically and engage politically.

Previously, Ms. Martinez Garcel served as the vice president of the New York State Health Foundation (NYSHealth). As a founding staff member, she was a key advisor to the president and helped establish the foundation as a resource for policy makers and community leaders across the state. She also played a central role in developing the foundation's program areas and developing partnerships with national and local foundations. Prior to joining NYSHealth, she served as the executive director of community voices in New York City. During her tenure, she developed, evaluated, and expanded programs to improve the health and quality of care for vulnerable populations.

Ms. Martinez Garcel has also served as a National Institutes of Health fellow for the Merida Department of Public Health in Yucatan, Mexico, a faculty member for the Social Science Department of the Borough of Manhattan Community College, and an adjunct professor at the New York University Global Institute of Public Health. She has been appointed to several boards, including the Institute for Civic Leadership, National Alliance on Mental Illness–NYC Metro, and Grantmakers in Health. She currently serves on the KQED Community Advisory Panel and co-chairs the National Latino Funds Alliance. Ms. Martinez Garcel has published extensively on issues related to health equity, vulnerable populations, and community health workers. She holds an M.P.H. from Columbia University and a B.S. from Cornell University.

Phyllis D. Meadows, Ph.D., R.N., M.S.N., is a senior fellow in the Health Program of The Kresge Foundation. She engages in all levels of grantmaking activity. Since joining The Kresge Foundation in 2009, she has advised the health team on the development of its overall strategic direction and provided leadership in the design and implementation of grantmaking initiatives and projects. Dr. Meadows also has coached team members and created linkages to national organizations and experts in the health field. In addition, she regularly reviews grant proposals, aids prospective grantees in preparing funding requests, and provides health-related expertise.

Dr. Meadows's 30-year career spans the nursing, public health, academic, and philanthropic sectors. She is an associate dean for practice at the University of Michigan's School of Public Health and has lectured at the Wayne State University School of Nursing, the Oakland University School of Nursing, and Marygrove College. From 2004 to 2009, Dr. Meadows served as the deputy director, director, and public health officer at the Detroit Department of Health and Wellness Promotion. In the early 1990s, she traveled abroad as a Kellogg International Leadership Fellow and subsequently joined the W.K. Kellogg Foundation as a program director. She also served as the director of nursing for The Medical Team–Michigan.

José Montero, M.D., M.P.H., M.S., serves as the deputy director of the Centers for Disease Control and Prevention (CDC) and as the director of CDC's Office for State, Tribal, Local, and Territorial Support, and is responsible for overseeing support to U.S. health departments, tribal nations, and insular areas. He oversees key activities and technical assistance designed to improve the public health system's capacity and performance in an era of health reform. Previously, Dr. Montero served as the vice president of population health and health system integration at Cheshire Medical Center/Dartmouth-Hitchcock Keene. In that capacity, he helped the health care system advance its Healthy Monadnock population health strategy. Key components of this process were improved partnerships with all organizations engaged in addressing social determinants of health for the population served and development of a sustainability pathway for the region's population health strategy. For 7 years, Dr. Montero served as the director of the Division of Public Health Services at the New Hampshire Department of Health and Human Services. In that role, he led the delivery of high-quality, evidence-based services and prompt response to public health threats and emerging issues in the state. Dr. Montero holds an M.D. from the Universidad Nacional de Colombia. He specialized in family medicine and completed his residency at the Universidad del Valle in Cali, Colombia. He also holds an epidemiology degree from Pontificia Universidad Javeriana in Bogotá, Colombia, and a master's degree in health care delivery science from Dartmouth College.

Von D. Nguyen, M.D., M.P.H., is the vice president of clinical operations and innovations at the Blue Cross and Blue Shield of North Carolina.

Previously, Dr. Nguyen served as the acting associate director for policy at the Centers for Disease Control and Prevention (CDC). In that capacity, he supported the policy agenda across CDC and manages CDC's efforts to promote collaboration between the public health and health care delivery systems. Prior to joining CDC, Dr. Nguyen worked at the Center for Medicare & Medicaid Innovation on the State Innovation Models, Prevention, and Population Health projects, as well as the larger Health Care Delivery System Reform agenda. He is a primary care provider who practiced at a federally qualified health center prior to entering federal service. In addition to his experience in public health and health care delivery, Dr. Nguyen has worked as a management consultant for Fortune 500 companies, a medical underwriter for health insurance companies, and a medical director for Doctors Without Borders.

Ziad Obermeyer, M.D., M.Phil., is the Blue Cross of California Distinguished Associate Professor of Health Policy and Management at the University of California, Berkeley, School of Public Health where he does research at the intersection of machine learning, medicine, and health policy. He was previously an assistant professor at Harvard Medical School, where he received the Early Independence Award, the National Institutes of Health's most prestigious award for exceptional junior scientists. Dr. Obermeyer continues to practice emergency medicine in underserved parts of the United States. Prior to his career in medicine, he worked as a consultant to pharmaceutical and global health clients at McKinsey & Co. in New Jersey, Geneva, and Tokyo.

Alison Omens, M.P.A., is the chief strategy officer at JUST Capital. She is responsible for setting and implementing strategy to achieve mission impact for the organization. Her work includes overseeing programs, revenue, partnerships, development, and strategic engagement with companies, investors, foundations, and nonprofits. She has orchestrated program collaborations with BlackRock, The Aspen Institute, Harvard Business School, and others.

Ms. Omens was most recently the advisor for private-sector engagement to U.S. Secretary of Labor Tom Perez, where she managed the inclusive capitalism strategy for the secretary and with the White House. She was also responsible for engagement on the department's future-of-work efforts and its environmental, social, and governance investing guidance. Previously, she was the vice president at outreach strategies, an environmental strategic communications firm, and the director of media outreach for the AFL-CIO.

Ms. Omens is on the board of directors of JobsFirstNYC, which expands opportunities for out-of-work and out-of-school youth. She is on the advisory councils of NextGen Chamber, a business organization for millennial business owners, and LitWorld, which promotes youth literacy through storytelling. She is also the co-founder of Smash Squad, a network for women focused on doing well by doing good. Ms. Omens received her M.P.A. from the Harvard Kennedy School and her B.A. from Scripps College.

Chris Parker, M.P.H., M.B.B.S., is a research assistant professor in the dean's Office of the Andrew Young School of Policy Studies and the director of global and population health at the Georgia Health Policy Center. He holds a leadership role in many of the center's projects related to public health and program evaluation. His areas of expertise include strategic planning and evaluation, with a particular interest in projects that link population health and health care.

Mr. Parker is a skilled facilitator who has guided a significant number of multisectoral, state, and local organizational strategic and evaluation plans. He is the co-principal investigator for Bridging for Health: Improving Community Health through Innovations in Financing, sponsored by the Robert Wood Johnson Foundation. He also leads the center's growing health care workforce portfolio with a focus on Georgia's primary care assets to address gaps in light of the Patient Protection and Affordable Care Act, as well as the center's work on community health needs assessments. As a trained family physician who has worked with underserved populations and faith-based organizations, Mr. Parker brings his clinical and community linked experiences to addressing current and long-standing public health issues.

Mary A. Pittman, Dr.P.H., is the chief executive officer and president of the Public Health Institute (PHI), a U.S. and global nonprofit public health organization dedicated to improving health and equity through economic, social, and health care innovation. PHI has 700 employees around the globe working on critical public health issues. Dr. Pittman is a national leader in community health, addressing health inequities, promoting prevention, and quality of care. Her experience in public health and health care settings has made her an expert adviser in the field of population health and building healthier and more equitable communities and health systems.

During her tenure, PHI has been recognized three times as 1 of the 50 best nonprofit places to work in the nation. Dr. Pittman served for 6 years on the National Academies of Sciences, Engineering, and Medicine's Roundtable on Population Health Improvement, and the Healthy People 2030 advisory committee to the Secretary of the U.S. Department of Health and Human Services. Finally, she served as an expert advisor to the Let's Get Healthy California Task Force and numerous other advisory boards.

Jason Purnell, Ph.D., M.P.H., is the vice president of community health improvement for BJC HealthCare. He is responsible for the development, implementation, and evaluation of BJC's community health programs, and oversees BJC's connections with community-based programs that offer primary, secondary, and tertiary prevention for chronic conditions. Prior to joining BJC in August 2020, he spent more than a decade focused on health equity and social determinants of health as a faculty member in the Brown School at Washington University in St. Louis, where he retains an appointment as an associate professor.

Dr. Purnell is the founding director of Health Equity Works (formerly For the Sake of All), a research-based initiative that translates data and research on the social determinants of health into engaging products to accelerate community action. He, his team, and collaborators have been responsible for raising awareness and facilitating action on issues ranging from school health to affordable housing in the St. Louis region and beyond.

A native of St. Louis, Dr. Purnell graduated magna cum laude from Harvard University, with a bachelor's degree in government and philosophy. His doctoral degree in counseling psychology is from The Ohio State University, and his M.P.H. is from the University of Rochester School of Medicine and Dentistry.

He serves as a member of the Roundtable on Population Health Improvement of the National Academies of Sciences, Engineering, and Medicine; as the chair of the steering committee of the COVID-19 Regional Response Team, which he helped to establish; and on the board of the Show-Me School-Based Health Alliance, which grew out of a Health Equity Works working group on school-based health centers.

Soma Saha, M.D., M.S., is the founder and executive lead of well-being and equity in the World (WE in the World). Dr. Saha has dedicated her career to improving health, well-being, and equity through the development of thriving people, organizations, and communities. She has worked as a primary care internist and a pediatrician in the safety net and a global public health practitioner for more than 20 years. She has witnessed and demonstrated sustainable transformation in human and community flourishing around the world.

Dr. Saha is also the executive lead of the Well Being In the Nation (WIN) Network, which works to advance intergenerational well-being and equity. She continues to serve as a faculty member at Harvard Medical School and the Institute for Healthcare Improvement. Over the past 5 years, as the vice president at the Institute for Healthcare Improvement, Dr. Saha founded and led the 100 Million Healthier Lives (100MLives) initiative, which brought together more than 1,850 partners in more than 30 countries reaching more than 500 million people to improve health, well-being, and equity. She and her team at WE in the World continue to advance and scale the frameworks, tools, and outcomes from this initiative as a core implementation partner in 100MLives.

Previously, Dr. Saha served as the vice president of Patient-Centered Medical Home Development at the Cambridge Health Alliance (CHA), where she co-led a transformation that improved health outcomes for a safety net population above the national 90th percentile, improved joy and meaning of work for the workforce, and reduced medical expense by 10 percent. She served as the president of the medical staff of Cambridge Health Alliance, as well as the founding medical director of the CHA Revere Family Health Center and the Whidden Hospitalist Service, leading to substantial improvements in access, experience, quality, and cost for safety net patients.

In 2012, Dr. Saha was recognized as 1 of 10 inaugural Robert Wood Johnson Foundation Young Leaders for her contributions to improving the health of the nation. She has consulted with leaders from across the world, including Australia, Brazil, Denmark, Guyana, Singapore, Sweden, Tunisia, and the United Kingdom. She has appeared on a panel with the Dalai Lama, keynoted conferences around the world, had her work featured by Sanjay Gupta, and appeared on the Katie Couric Show, PBS, and CNN. In 2016 she was elected as a Leading Causes of Life Global Fellow.

Joshua M. Sharfstein, M.D., is the vice dean for public health practice and community engagement and a professor of the practice in health policy and management at the Johns Hopkins Bloomberg School of Public Health. He is also the director of the Bloomberg American Health Initiative. Previously, Dr. Sharfstein served as the secretary of the Maryland Department of Health and Mental Hygiene, the principal deputy commissioner of the U.S. Food and Drug Administration, and the health commissioner of the City of Baltimore. In these positions, he pursued creative solutions to long-standing challenges, including drug overdose deaths, infant mortality, unsafe consumer products, and school failure. He is an elected member of the National Academy of Medicine and the National Academy of Public Administration.

Marion Standish, M.A., J.D., is the senior vice president of Enterprise Programs at The California Endowment (TCE). She joined TCE with an extensive legal and philanthropic background. As the senior vice president of Enterprise Programs, she is responsible for managing resources that will support collaboration and alignment across all TCE departments to achieve TCE's mission and Building Health Communities goals and outcomes. Dr. Standish leads multiple philanthropic partnerships, provides strategic guidance to Impact Investing activities, and works closely with TCE's chief learning officer to achieve organizational goals. Dr. Standish serves as the lead officer for the Endowment with the Partnership for a Healthier America and the National Convergence Partnership, and she previously served as the lead officer for First Lady Michelle Obama's Let's Move Initiative and California's Let's Get Healthy effort.

Previously, Dr. Standish was the senior advisor to the president of TCE and the director of community health, where she oversaw multiple grantmaking initiatives focused on transforming communities to reduce inequities and improving health. She played a key role in developing and implementing many TCE signature initiatives, including the Partnership for the Public's Health, Community Action to Fight Asthma, and Healthy Eating Active Communities. Before joining TCE, Dr. Standish was the founder and the director of California Food Policy Advocates (CFPA), a statewide nutrition and health research and advocacy organization focusing on access to nutritious food for low-income families. Before launching CFPA, she served as the director of the California Rural Legal Assistance Foundation, a statewide advocacy organization focusing on health, education, and labor issues facing farmworkers and the rural poor. She began her career as a staff attorney with California Rural Legal Assistance, a federally funded legal services program. Dr. Standish received her J.D. from the University of San Francisco School of Law and both her M.A. and undergraduate degrees from New York University.

Monica Valdes Lupi, J.D., M.P.H., joined The Kresge Foundation as the managing director for health programs in September 2020. With more than 20 years of experience in public health, Ms. Valdes Lupi leads the Health Team in building equity-focused systems of health that create opportunities for all people to achieve well-being. Prior to joining The Kresge Foundation, she was the senior fellow for the de Beaumont Foundation, where she served as an advisor to amplify and accelerate policy initiatives aimed at developing and advancing a health agenda on critical public health issues such as tobacco control, racial justice, and health equity. Ms. Valdes Lupi also worked as a senior advisor to the Centers for Disease Control and Prevention Foundation (CDCF) in its COVID-19 efforts. In this role, she helped guide activities aimed at quickly identifying and supporting gaps and needs among state and local health departments in their response and recovery activities. Working alongside CDCF's leadership team, Ms. Valdes Lupi was particularly focused on building support for vulnerable populations such as the homeless, older adults, and Black and Latinx communities. She has extensive governmental public health experience as the executive director of the Boston Public Health Commission, the local health department for the City of Boston, and also as the deputy commissioner for the Massachusetts Department of Public Health. She has also led national efforts through her role as chief program officer for health systems transformation at the Association of State and Territorial Health Officials.

Stella Whitney-West, M.B.A., is the chief executive officer of NorthPoint Health & Wellness Center, a federally qualified health center that serves more than 25,000 residents in North Minneapolis and Hennepin County with comprehensive medical, dental, and behavioral health care. Prior to her appointment, she served as the chief operating officer for North-Point's Human Services. Her background includes more than two decades of experience working with governance and policy boards of nonprofit organizations as well as extensive senior management experience in the Twin Cities nonprofit community.

She has an M.B.A. from the University of St. Thomas and a B.S. in biology from the University of Minnesota. Ms. Whitney-West serves on the Twin Cities Local Initiatives Support Corporation Advisory Board and as a member of the board of directors for Stratis Health and Urban Home Works. She is currently the board president for the Minnesota Association of Community Health Centers.